Activism and Marginalization in the AIDS Crisis

D0168915

Activism
and Marginalization
in the AIDS Crisis

Michael A. Hallett, PhD
Editor

Activism and Marginalization in the AIDS Crisis, edited by Michael A. Hallett, was simultaneously issued by The Haworth Press, Inc., under the same title, as a special issue of *Journal of Homosexuality,* Volume 32, Numbers 3/4, 1997, John P. De Cecco, Editor.

Harrington Park Press
An Imprint of
The Haworth Press, Inc.
New York • London

ISBN 1-56023-090-8

Published by

Harrington Park Press, 10 Alice Street, Binghamton, NY 13904-1580 USA

Harrington Park Press is an Imprint of the Haworth Press, Inc., 10 Alice Street, Binghamton, NY 13904-1580 USA.

Activism and Marginalization in the AIDS Crisis has also been published as *Journal of Homosexuality*, Volume 32, Numbers 3/4 1997.

Cover design by Marylouise E. Doyle

Library of Congress Cataloging-in-Publication Data

Activism and marginalization in the AIDS crisis / Michael A. Hallett, editor.
    p. cm.
    Includes bibliographical references and index.
    ISBN 0-7890-0004-0 (THP : alk. paper). – ISBN 1-56023-090-8 (HPP : alk. paper)
    1. AIDS (Disease)–Social aspects–United States. 2. Political activists–United States. 3. AIDS (Disease) in mass media–United States. I. Hallett, Michael A.
RA644.A25A277 1997
362.1'969792'00973–dc21
                                   97-700
                                    CIP

For Karin

I believe you would have made it without me;
I could never have made it without you.

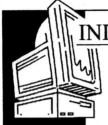

INDEXING & ABSTRACTING

Contributions to this publication are selectively indexed or abstracted in print, electronic, online, or CD-ROM version(s) of the reference tools and information services listed below. This list is current as of the copyright date of this publication. See the end of this section for additional notes.

- *Abstracts in Anthropology*, Baywood Publishing Company, 26 Austin Avenue, P.O. Box 337, Amityville, NY 11701

- *Abstracts of Research in Pastoral Care & Counseling*, Loyola College, 7135 Minstrel Way, Suite 101, Columbia, MD 21045

- *Academic Abstracts/CD-ROM*, EBSCO Publishing Editorial Department, P.O. Box 590, Ipswich, MA 01938-0590

- *Academic Search: database of 2,000 selected academic serials, updated monthly,* EBSCO Publishing, 83 Pine Street, Peabody, MA 01960

- *Alternative Press Index,* Alternative Press Center, Inc., P.O. Box 33109, Baltimore, MD 21218-0401

- *Applied Social Sciences Index & Abstracts (ASSIA) (Online: ASSI via Data-Star) (CD-Rom: ASSIA Plus)*, Bowker- Saur Limited, Maypole House, Maypole Road, East Grinstead, West Sussex RH19 1HH England

- *Book Review Index,* Gale Research, Inc., P.O. Box 2867, Detroit, MI 48231

- *Cambridge Scientific Abstracts*, *Risk Abstracts*, Environmental Routenet (accessed via INTERNET), 7200 Wisconsin Avenue, #601, Bethesda, MD 20814

- *CNPIEC Reference Guide: Chinese National Directory of Foreign Periodicals,* P.O. Box 88, Beijing, People's Republic of China

- *Criminal Justice Abstracts*, Willow Tree Press, 15 Washington Street, 4th Floor, Newark NJ 07102

(continued)

- *Criminology, Penology and Police Science Abstracts*, Kugler Publications, P.O. Box 11188, 1001 GD-Amsterdam, The Netherlands

- *Current Contents/Clinical Medicine/Life Sciences (CC: CM/LS) (weekly Table of Contents Service), and* Social Science Citation Index. *Articles also searchable through* Social SciSearch, *ISI's online database and in ISI's* Research Alert *current awareness service,* Institute for Scientific Information, 3501 Market Street, Philadelphia, PA 19104-3302

- *Digest of Neurology and Psychiatry,* The Institute of Living, 400 Washington Street, Hartford, CT 06106

- *Excerpta Medica/Secondary Publishing Division*, Elsevier Science, Inc., Secondary Publishing Division, 655 Avenue of the Americas, New York, NY 10010

- *Expanded Academic Index*, Information Access Company, 362 Lakeside Drive, Forest City, CA 94404

- *Family Life Educator "Abstracts Section,"* ETR Associates, P.O. Box 1830, Santa Cruz, CA 95061-1830

- *Family Studies Database (online and CD/ROM)*, National Information Services Corporation, 306 East Baltimore Pike, 2nd Floor, Media, PA 19063

- *Family Violence & Sexual Assault Bulletin*, Family Violence & Sexual Assault Institute, 1121 East South East Loop 323, Suite 130, Tyler, TX 75701

- *Higher Education Abstracts,* The Claremont Graduate School, 231 East Tenth Street, Claremont, CA 91711

- *HOMODOK/"Relevant" Bibliographic database, Documentation Centre for Gay & Lesbian Studies, University of Amsterdam (selective printed abstracts in "Homologie" and bibliographic computer databases covering cultural, historical, social and political aspects of gay & lesbian topics),* % HOMODOK-ILGA Archive, O.Z. Achterburgwal 185, NL-1012 DK Amsterdam, The Netherlands

(continued)

- *IBZ International Bibliography of Periodical Literature*, Zeller Verlag GmbH & Co., P.O.B. 1949, d-49009 Osnabruck, Germany

- *Index Medicus*, National Library of Medicine, 8600 Rockville Pike, Bethesda, MD 20894

- *Index to Periodical Articles Related to Law*, University of Texas, 727 East 26th Street, Austin, TX 78705

- *INTERNET ACCESS (& additional networks) Bulletin Board for Libraries ("BUBL"), coverage of information resources on INTERNET, JANET, and other networks.*
  - JANET X.29: UK.AC.BATH.BUBL or 00006012101300
  - TELNET: BUBL.BATH.AC.UK or 138.38.32.45 login 'bubl'
  - Gopher: BUBL.BATH.AC.UK (138.32.32.45). Port 7070
  - World Wide Web: http: / / www.bubl.bath.ac.uk./BUBL/ home.html
  - NISSWAIS: telnetniss.ac.uk (for the NISS gateway)
  The Andersonian Library, Curran Building, 101 St. James Road, Glasgow G4 ONS, Scotland

- *Leeds Medical Information*, University of Leeds, Leeds LS2 9JT, United Kingdom

- *MasterFILE: updated database from EBSCO Publishing,* 83 Pine Street, Peabody, MA 01960

- *Mental Health Abstracts (online through DIALOG)*, IFI/Plenum Data Company, 3202 Kirkwood Highway, Wilmington, DE 19808

- *MLA International Bibliography,* Modern Language Association of America, 10 Astor Place, New York, NY 10003

- *PASCAL International Bibliography T205: Sciences de l'information Documentation*, INIST/CNRS-Service Gestion des Documents Primaires, 2, allée du Parc de Brabois, F-54514 Vandoeuvre-les-Nancy, Cedex, France

- *Periodical Abstracts, Research I (general and basic reference indexing and abstracting data-base from University Micro-films International (UMI), 300 North Zeeb Road, P.O. Box 1346, Ann Arbor, MI 48106-1346)*, UMI Data Courier, P.O. Box 32770, Louisville, KY 40232-2770

(continued)

- *Periodical Abstracts, Research II (broad coverage indexing and abstracting data-base from University Microfilms International (UMI), 300 North Zeeb Road, P.O. Box 1346, Ann Arbor, MI 48106-1346)*, UMI Data Courier, P.O. Box 32770, Louisville, KY 40232-2770

- *PsychNet*, PsychNet Inc., P.O. Box 369, Georgetown, CO 80444

- *Public Affairs Information Bulletin (PAIS)*, Public Affairs Information Service, Inc., 521 West 43rd Street, New York, NY 10036-4396

- *Religion Index One: Periodicals, the index to Book Reviews in Religion, Religion Indexes: RIO/RIT/IBRR 1975- on CD/ROM,* American Theological Library Association, 820 Church Street, 3rd Floor, Evanston, IL 60201
  - E-mail: atla@atla.com
  - WWW: http://atla.library.vanderbilt.edu/atla/home.html

- *Sage Family Studies Abstracts (SFSA),* Sage Publications, Inc., 2455 Teller Road, Newbury Park, CA 91320

- *Social Planning/Policy & Development Abstracts (SOPODA)*, Sociological Abstracts, Inc., P.O. Box 22206, San Diego, CA 92192-0206

- *Social Sciences Index (from Volume 1 & continuing)*, The H.W. Wilson Company, 950 University Avenue, Bronx, NY 10452

- *Social Science Source: coverage of 400 journals in the social sciences area; updated monthly,* EBSCO Publishing, 83 Pine Street, P.O. Box 2250, Peabody, MA 01960-7250

- *Social Work Abstracts*, National Association of Social Workers, 750 First Street NW, 8th Floor, Washington, DC 20002

- *Sociological Abstracts (SA)*, Sociological Abstracts, Inc., P.O. Box 22206, San Diego, CA 92192-0206

- *Studies on Women Abstracts*, Carfax Publishing Company, P.O. Box 25, Abingdon, Oxfordshire OXI4 3UE, United Kingdom

- *Violence and Abuse Abstracts: A Review of Current Literature on Interpersonal Violence (VAA),* Sage Publications, Inc., 2455 Teller Road, Newbury Park, CA 91320

Book reviews are selectively excerpted by the Guide to Professional Literature of the Journal of Academic Librarianship.

SPECIAL BIBLIOGRAPHIC NOTES

related to special journal issues (separates)
and indexing/abstracting

☐ indexing/abstracting services in this list will also cover material in any "separate" that is co-published simultaneously with Haworth's special thematic journal issue or DocuSerial. Indexing/abstracting usually covers material at the article/chapter level.

☐ monographic co-editions are intended for either non-subscribers or libraries which intend to purchase a second copy for their circulating collections.

☐ monographic co-editions are reported to all jobbers/wholesalers/approval plans. The source journal is listed as the "series" to assist the prevention of duplicate purchasing in the same manner utilized for books-in-series.

☐ to facilitate user/access services all indexing/abstracting services are encouraged to utilize the co-indexing entry note indicated at the bottom of the first page of each article/chapter/contribution.

☐ this is intended to assist a library user of any reference tool (whether print, electronic, online, or CD-ROM) to locate the monographic version if the library has purchased this version but not a subscription to the source journal.

☐ individual articles/chapters in any Haworth publication are also available through the Haworth Document Delivery Services (HDDS).

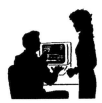

CONTENTS

ABOUT THE EDITOR

Michael A. Hallett, PhD, is Assistant Professor of Criminal Justice Administration at Middle Tennessee State University. Dr. Hallett's work explores mediated presentations of social issues and the means by which institutions subvert and transform public discourse. His recent publications appear in the *International Journal of Public Administration, Evaluation & Program Planning, Peace Review*, and the *American Journal of Police*. Professor Hallett received his doctorate from the School of Justice Studies at Arizona State University.

Activism and Marginalization in the AIDS Crisis

ACKNOWLEDGMENTS

In the course of a project like this, many debts are incurred. First, I wish to acknowledge a special debt to Professor Michael Musheno, School of Justice Studies, Arizona State University, who brought me into his research on HIV/AIDS during my doctoral candidacy at Arizona State. While providing constructive criticism on this and other work, Professor Musheno constantly seeks (and succeeds) to push me further. For this I am deeply grateful.

Each of the authors contributing to this collection also gave me several helpful critiques and shared their unique insights. In particular, Professor Dion Dennis provided supportive criticism and (as always) earnest friendship.

In addition to these debts, I owe debts of gratitude to Professor John DeCecco, Editor of the *Journal of Homosexuality*, whose consistent support allowed me to focus and work; Stephanie Kane, who provided insightful criticism; and finally, Dean Anne Schneider, Arizona State University, who provided myself and several of my co-authors with reprints of her work and valuable comments on our own.

Of course, responsibility for any weaknesses or flaws in this collection remains with me.

M. H.

Foreword

Nearly ten years ago Randy Shilts published *And the Band Played On* (1987), a brilliant and iconoclastic indictment of the institutional response of the medical profession, the federal and state medical agencies and Federal medical research Institutes, and politicians to the emergent AIDS epidemic. Very attentive to factual and personal nuance, clever in conception (the life events of a handful of fated activists were woven into a narrative outlining the medical mystery of the disease and patterns of insensitive, hesitant governmental response), painfully honest and lucid, the book was hailed, a best-seller, and widely honored. It went largely ignored by social scientists. Responses to this book were a harbinger of future developments outlined in this skillfully edited and welcome collection assembled and introduced by Michael Hallett. I shall try in this brief essay to illuminate some themes in the social drama of AIDS.

Unfortunately, Randy Shilts, like most of his friends who were in slightly modified form the protagonists in his book, is dead of AIDS. He courageously carried on after being diagnosed (as his first book was published to rave reviews) and managed to complete his second book on homosexuals in the military. Susan Sontag, in her somewhat pretentious *AIDS and Its Metaphors* (1989), drawing on literary criticism and history, approached the AIDS problem phenomenologically, examining at the level of meaning, while interpolating the representations of the disease with patterns of politics and social structure. Shilts embedded his examining of the meaning of the disease within the narratives of medical research and political indifference. These two books enacted the opening

[Haworth co-indexing entry note]: "Foreword." Manning, P. K. Co-published simultaneously in *The Journal of Homosexuality* (The Haworth Press, Inc.) Vol. 32, No. 3/4, 1997, pp. xxi-xxviii; and: *Activism and Marginalization in the AIDS Crisis* (ed: Michael A. Hallett) The Haworth Press, Inc., 1997, pp. xvii-xxiv; and: *Activism and Marginalization in the AIDS Crisis* (ed: Michael A. Hallett) Harrington Park Press, an imprint of The Haworth Press, Inc., 1997, pp. xv-xxii. Single or multiple copies of this article are available for a fee from The Haworth Document Delivery Service [1-800-342-9678, 9:00 a.m. - 5:00 p.m. (EST). E-mail address: getinfo@haworth.com].

scenes of a still-unfolding social drama of meaning and authority. They encourage us to analyze the unfolding character of AIDS as a secular drama Act I. The opening scene is played out by medical researchers. In the late eighties, medical researchers sought to tease out the genetic, biochemical, and physiological mechanisms by which AIDS was contracted and transmitted, to differentiate stages in the natural history of the disease, and to describe its course in the medical language of etiology, diagnosis, prognosis, and therapy. Almost from the outset, the central players who defined the terms of reference were specialist medical doctors–epidemiologists at the Centers for Disease Control, Biochemists at NIH, and geneticists in Paris–all of whom focused on the disease as a biomedical phenomenon. It was seen as chronic, debilitating disease produced by chemical and biochemical forces represented in cells in the immunological system. Admittedly, it had psycho-social sequelae. These were distinguished from "the disease," but the illness, symbolizing the disease and its social, cultural, and behavioral components, remained secondary to the authorities.

The second scene reveals the results of scene one. The biomedical strategy of research created a series of anomalies, some of which are discussed in papers in this collection. It defined the disease as a biological entity which at the time appeared to stand tantalizingly outside known medical modes of prevention, treatment, and cure and firmly located the cause, treatment, and cure (almost entirely) within the biomedical realm. It defined prevention and cure biochemically. I implied above, this strategy isolated the social meanings of the disease and disconnected them from its ostensive biomedical nature. It is an illness known to arise and spread within a context that made it analogous to other morally dubious and fearful diseases. Some felt it was a kind of plague visited upon sinners. To others, the disease communicated a double-coded message: it was dreaded and dreadful both to individual and to society. By the mid-eighties it was extracting very high costs, especially among the young and talented. Extrapolations, difficult to produce because of the long and variable dormant phase, predicted millions of victims within ten years.

Unfortunately, this definition suppressed attention to the illness–the social, psychological and psychiatric dimensions–and to the psycho-social contexts within which the disease appeared and is transmitted. The combination of biomedical focus and moral metaphors made it possible for large cities like New York to withhold investment of human resources from research and care options and for insurance companies to eschew responsibility or cancel coverage. The victims of AIDS were morally differentiated. Ironically, those who were medical victims—as a result of familial transmission, mismanagement of blood supplies or failed screening of transfusions, or as a result of accidents at work (surgeons for example), were made martyrs. Those whose disease was sexually transmitted were stigmatized.

ACT II

The second act shows the consequences of the dramatic actions in Act I. This dramaturgical strategy of (biomedical) definition left implicit, as with all sexually transmitted diseases, the bases for making moral judgements. Are those with AIDS "victims," "survivors," "patients," "sinners," and do they deserve pity, reprobation, condemnation, tolerance, prayers, education, rehabilitation (and conversion), or punishment? What do they owe society and what does society, writ large, require or owe them? Clearly, a political debate about the appropriate metaphor within which to discuss the disease had real, fateful consequences.

Is AIDS "deviance" to be punished? Is it a disease to be treated? Is it a label or vehicle for avoiding feeling, compassion, and concern? Is the spread of AIDS a moral plague that threatens to erode and transgress social boundaries? Internationally, nations differed in their patterns of response including isolation, extrusion and exclusion, treatment, punishment, and attempts to expel. All this suggests that the biomedical focus had a not-insignificant effect upon the social construction of the illness. We live within our created meanings, but we do not always have a meaningful role in creating them.

ACT III

Public responses to medical and political definitions. Each definition of AIDS employs a metaphor to establish the nature and logic of the disease. When thinking metaphorically or analogically, we think about one thing in terms of another. The terms, disease, plague, epidemic, moral panic, crime, deviance, life-style tariff, are all partial portraits of subtle multi-leveled processes that affect biological (neurological, biochemical, physiological, and anatomical) social and psycho-social levels of functioning. It is seen best in a bio-psychosocial model. These metaphoric formulations shape the rhetoric, the logic of words, the logomachy of the AIDS drama. According to Kenneth Burke (1970), the logic of words creates a hierarchy of sacrifice and redemption, for how as well as why something is called establishes action choices. Words construct the sets within which we act out our fates. Clearly, the rhetorics that order and stratify the meanings of AIDS have limited policy efforts and public expectations. Consider these options. If a person is morally responsible and accountable, deviant, wandering from the conventional path, he or she requires punishment. If a person is merely ignorant, innocent of intention, he or she might be a candidate for education or rehabilitation, or ordered to make restitution to society. If a person contracts a disease, moral opprobrium is obviated, and treatment ensues. One is not seen as morally responsible for cancer, pneumonia, or a congenitally malfunctioning heart. If, through no fault of one's own, one becomes diseased as a result of others' malfeasance, then society owes the victim. Someone else is to blame and should compensate the innocent party. These rhetorics of responsibility carry the shadows of morality and blame with them. Depending on the metaphor and the logomachy it connotes, social policies and actions will vary. However, as chapters by Hallett and Cannella and Dion Dennis show, the media have an active, creative, intentional, and dramatic effect on the drama and crisis of AIDS through their gatekeeping function, use of metaphor and selective story lines, and concern for maintaining circulation and viewers.

Clearly, as chapters on AIDS information and citizens' groups in this volume show, labels and rhetorics are confused and confounded in the case of AIDS. We blame the victim, condemn the sick, isolate and stigmatize the diseased, and withhold care and compromise already limited welfare efforts. This state of affairs, an axial consequence of definitional work, reflects variously upon American society. Our Puritan-sourced ambivalence toward pleasure and sexual pleasure (especially outside marriage) leads to a focus on individuals and stigmatization and marginalization of "sexual deviants." Our fragmented and underdeveloped welfare system, the least capacious and generous in the industrialized world, withholds care and concern from the poor and unemployed, and locates the cause of poverty and unemployment in already disadvantaged individuals. Our medical care system, the least efficient (about 15% is spent in the administration and profit-taking by insurance companies) and most top-heavy of the industrialized world, treats acute and chronic illness with high technology while dehumanizing and prolonging life. The current anti-government mood encourages further cuts in social services, education, and medical research. As Hallett demonstrates in his essay, AIDS has been shamefully neglected, for these reasons as well as for its association with sexually transmitted diseases and a few of the variety of homosexual lifestyles, and other condemned lifestyles.

An irony in this drama, as Shilts shows, is that the gay community (being a misnomer in this regard), was not of one mind with regard to the proper response to AIDS. Some argued against preventive public health measures such as closing the bath houses in San Francisco; some argued for abstinence and altered lifestyles; some wished to focus attention on AIDS victims, soliciting support within the entertainment industry (symbolized by wearing small red lapel ribbons); others, such as Shilts himself, urged active political campaigns to educate the public and correct the worst and most stigmatizing myths. In the end, many key players and organizations disappeared; the AIDS Commission under Reagan faded; the political pressure in New York City, documented by Perrow and Guillen (1990), seemed to abate with little change in allocation for care facilities. Focus then turned to those rare, wealthy, and sophisticated people who had survived for several years after an HIV-positive diagnosis. Ervin Johnson was featured on the cover of *Newsweek* (January, 1996) when he announced he was returning to play professional basketball. Other notable survivors (mostly "innocent victims" as noted above) were featured in the *Newsweek* story. Newspaper reports in early 1996 have hopeful developments in biochemical processes that may insulate or diminish the risk of AIDS in some.

ACT IV

This dialectic in the definition of AIDS communicates powerfully about basic social processes. A strategy of labelling and selective differential attention to a complex, multifaceted matter such as "AIDS" (consider it now as a sign without a clear referent) arises, partially a result of media attention, partially as a result of the differential power of experts in problem. Each defines, and partially as a result of the varying capacity and resources of the labelled or "target group" to "fight back," the definitions may stick. Labelling, it is now well understood, is not a one-way process, but an ongoing struggle. The elevation and diminution of selected social groups and lifestyles associated in the public mind with the disease is joined by groups with a vested interest in the outcomes in a debate over the emergent primordial themes that will characterize political debate.

Underlying this social process is the material biological reality of the disease's processes and their overt symptomatic manifestations. Even if a "cure," or effective therapy, should be found soon, in the next few years, a large and ever-growing number of people will have suffered and died. It is unlikely that any discovered therapy will reverse the terrible, devastating effects of the multi-leveled processes associated with the disease. Nevertheless, the dialectic of blame and guilt, the labelling and extrusion of the ill and diseased, and counter-strategies of redefining the meanings of the disease will continue into the next century. Unfortunately, the disease spreads now among the powerless and disadvantaged, and remains linked to lifestyle questions—sexual preferences (including prostitution); addictions and choices of drugs; and access to medical care and social services. AIDS is a disease and an illness and a moral construct.

The political and moral debate over AIDS, its causes and possible treatments, carried on extensively and passionately in the mid-eighties, seemed to have died at some point in the early nineties. Yet, the outlines of this debate are reflected in the moral career of those with AIDS. My colleague, Betsy Cullum-Swan, interviewed in depth some eight young men diagnosed as HIV-positive in the mid-eighties (Cullum-Swan, 1987). Several are known to have died since. It seemed that an HIV-positive person had a career line that manifested several stages from ignorance and denial to questioning and worry, and finally of knowledge of being tested positive. Not all passed through all the stages, and some continued to deny the illness even after testing positive, but the stage notion seemed to order the experience. At the time, little was known of how long people might live while HIV-positive, and it was a depressing and depressed group who felt like living dead. Not all those interviewed responded to the knowledge in the same fashion; some worked at organizing their friendships, some regressed, others continued to study and work. Much more is unknown than known about the careers of persons with AIDS.

These papers show how the mass media and conventional wisdom have limited and constrained policy options. AIDS remains an ambiguous figure that enters and leaves the political stage, sometimes in the guise of debates about morality, sometimes about medical and social resources, and sometimes about the family and "family values." One way to marginalize a problem, as the authors of these chapters show, is to define it as a semi-visible subtext under another name, and to use allegories, code words, and metaphors to cloak it in mystery and obscurity. These analyses suggest further that even a Nobel Prize-winning medical breakthrough in etiology, treatment, or cure will little alter the moral and political rhetoric surrounding AIDS, and the burden of being unwilling players in social drama not of their choosing will continue to be shifted to those least able to cope with it.

Peter K. Manning, PhD
School of Criminal Justice
Department of Sociology
Michigan State University
February 29, 1996

LIST OF REFERENCES CITED

Burke, Kenneth. (1970). *The Rhetoric of Religion*. Berkeley: University of California Press.

Cullum-Swan, Betsy. (1987). "The AIDS Career . . . . ." presented to the Society for Symbolic Interaction, Stone Symposium, UCSF, San Francisco.

Perrow, Charles, and M. Guillen. (1990). *The AIDS Disaster: The Failure of Organizations in New York and the Nation*. New Haven: Yale University Press.

Shilts, Randy. (1987). *And the Band Played On: Politics, People and the AIDS Epidemic*. New York: St. Martins.

Sontag, Susan. (1989). *AIDS and Its Metaphors*. New York: Farrar, Straus and Giroux.

Public health authorities estimate that there are about 1 million people currently infected in the United States, many of them unrecognized carriers. Thus, even if all HIV transmission were to cease, the greatest impact of the epidemic would lie ahead. It is sometimes argued that rates of transmission have stabilized or even peaked in certain behavioral risk groups; this assessment may be premature, but even if it is accurate most symptomatic disease will manifest itself in the future. As a society we have yet to experience the full magnitude of this epidemic, whether it is measured in terms of total person-years of illness and disability, in terms of the economic and social costs of medical care and social service systems, or in terms of the absolute number of deaths.

Dr. Helena Brett-Smith, MD
Dr. Gerald Friedland, MD
1992

Power is the ability to have one's position heard.

Leslie Miller
"Claimsmaking from the Underside,"
in *Constructionist Controversies*

I'm here for you to save my life. Is that too political?

Ned Weeks

Introduction:
Activism and Marginalization
in the AIDS Crisis

Michael A. Hallett, PhD

Middle Tennessee State University

HOW WE "KNOW" WHAT WE "KNOW" ABOUT HIV: ON INSTITUTIONALLY-STRUCTURED EPISTEMOLOGIES OF AIDS

In perhaps the most widely-read cultural discussion about what HIV/AIDS "means," Susan Sontag laments the use of the "military metaphor" in understanding and fighting disease:

> AIDS marks a turning point in current attitudes toward illness and medicine, as well as toward sexuality and catastrophe. Medicine had been viewed as an age-old military campaign now nearing its final phase, leading to victory. The emergence of a new epidemic disease, when for several decades it had been confidently assumed that such calamities belonged to the past, has inevitably changed the status of medicine. The advent of AIDS makes it clear that the infectious diseases are far from conquered and their roster far from closed. (1989, p. 72)

Michael A. Hallett is Assistant Professor in the Department of Criminal Justice at Middle Tennessee State University.

[Haworth co-indexing entry note]: "Introduction: Activism and Marginalization in the AIDS Crisis." Hallett, Michael A. Co-published simultaneously in *Journal of Homosexuality* (The Haworth Press, Inc.) Vol. 32, No. 3/4, 1997, pp. 1-16; and: *Activism and Marginalization in the AIDS Crisis* (ed: Michael A. Hallett) The Haworth Press, Inc., 1997, pp. 1-16; and: *Activism and Marginalization in the AIDS Crisis* (ed: Michael A. Hallett) Harrington Park Press, an imprint of The Haworth Press, Inc., 1997, pp. 1-16. Single or multiple copies of this article are available for a fee from The Haworth Document Delivery Service [1-800-342-9678, 9:00 a.m. - 5:00 p.m. (EST). E-mail address: get info@haworth.com].

The readings in this volume collectively suggest that in addition to the disavowal of the military metaphor in the bio-medical sciences, for example, the advent of HIV-disease has also brought into question the utility of certain forms of "activism" as they relate to understanding and fighting the *social* impacts of disease.[1]

This volume is centrally concerned about the ways in which institutionally governed social constructions of HIV/AIDS affect policy. The thesis of this book is that an accounting of the power *institutional structures* have over the dominant social constructions of HIV-disease is fundamental to adequate forms of present and future AIDS activism. To understand the sui generis nature of HIV-related discourse, it is necessary to first account for the power of institutional structures (more below). The chapters of this volume demonstrate how–despite what is thought of as the "successful activism" of the past decade–the claims of the HIV-positive are *still* being ignored, still being marginalized, and still being administratively "handled" and exploited–as the plight of those who find themselves HIV-positive objectively worsens.[2]

This collection of essays specifically concerns itself with the ways in which (concrete) institutions, e.g., for-profit media corporations, prison administrations, federal and state government bureaucracies, Governor's AIDS Task Forces, and academic journals, have regularly employed and/or adulterated discourse about HIV/AIDS to serve–not the interests of the HIV-positive–but their own interests. The readings provide multiple accounts of institutional power working to govern public understanding of HIV-disease–with particular attention paid to the ways in which discourses promoted by institutional structures affect HIV-related policy.

On any given day, certainly for the past several years, Americans have encountered competing and often contradictory messages about the state and progression of the HIV/AIDS crisis (Bayer, 1989; Keniston, 1990; Kitzinger, 1990). These messages have had less to do with any "objective reality" about HIV-disease, than with the institutions propagating these messages in the first place (Cobb & Elder, 1972; Cobb et al., 1976). As a result, the general public has experienced a kind of institutionally governed "information overload" which must be sorted through and accounted for as future AIDS activist agendas emerge.

As we see it, the problem is that public (including "activist") discourse about HIV/AIDS is routinely sensationalized, watered down, shunted, and/or ignored altogether—*according to the configured interests of institutional structures* (Altheide & Snow, 1979; Thomas et al., 1987). The fight, this book contends, is no longer best understood as a monolithic battle against ambivalent and self-serving state bureaucracies that deny access to rights or benefits: it is better understood as a struggle against a *new condition of governance* in which *ensembles* of *institutional structures* (only some of which are "governmental") effectively seek to dominate the social construction of policy issues along lines advantageous to given sets of interests (Cobb & Elder, 1972). This, as we have seen with so many social problems, results in several competing kinds of "answers," all of which are conceptually amputated because they are founded upon merely rhetorical and institutionally self-serving presentations of social issues (Cobb et al., 1976; Hallett, 1994; Palumbo et al., 1994).

Institutional Structures Defined

The term "institutional structure," as utilized here, is that developed by George Thomas, John Meyer, Francisco Ramirez, and John Boli in their 1987 book *Institutional Structure: Constituting State, Society, and the Individual:*

> By *institution* we mean a set of cultural rules that give generalized meaning to social activity and regulate it in a patterned way. (p. 37)

Institutional structures, then, are groupings engaged in and *defined by* the production of various "truths" which sustain them. In this sense, given sufficient institutional power, an "activist" group could certainly become an "institutional structure." *Institutional power* may be defined as the capacity to regulate, constrain, and disseminate versions of "truth" (especially Miller, 1993; Guba & Lincoln, 1989; Ericson et al., 1989).

As revealed by these readings, however, "HIV-activist" groups have been out-maneuvered when it comes to the production and dissemination of various "truths" about HIV/AIDS by institutional structures more deeply steeped in social legitimacy than groups like ACT UP, for example, and by institutional structures having superior capacity for message dissemination (Kramer, 1992; Stipp & Kerr, 1989; Watney, 1989).[3]

A central concern of our analysis is the way institutional structures create and legitimize social entities that are seen as "actors." That is, institutionalized cultural rules define the meaning and identity of the individual and the patterns of appropriate economic, political, and cultural activity engaged in by those individuals. They similarly constitute the purposes and legitimacy of organizations, professions, interest groups, and states, while delineating lines of activity appropriate to these entities (Thomas et al., pp. 12-13).

Institutionalization, then, involves the processes that make such sets of rules seem natural and taken for granted while eliminating alternative interpretations and regulations (Thomas et al., p. 37).

Here, it is useful to distinguish between what might be called "concrete" institutional structures (e.g., health insurance bureaucracies, governmental subcommittees, prison administrations, or court systems) and what post-modernists call "new" institutions (the discourses that *sustain* concrete institutions). Here, these two forms are seen as distinguishable but inseparable. Writes Foucault with regard to discourse:

> In a society such as ours, but basically in any society, there are manifold relations of power which permeate, characterize and constitute the social body, and these relations of power cannot themselves be established, consolidated nor implemented without the production, accumulation, circulation, and functioning of a discourse. There can be no possible exercise of power without a certain economy of discourses of truth which operates through and on the basis of this association. We are subject to the production of truth through power and we cannot exercise power except through the production of truth. (1979, p. 93)

This volume came about as the result of a dialogue about activism I engaged in with editors at the *Journal of Homosexuality,* after an article I had submitted to that journal was accepted for publication. The article pointed to the relative failure of activists to achieve a highly visible and sustained HIV-positive voice in the mainstream press (see chapter 2). My co-author (a medical reporter for a major mainstream newspaper) and I argued that despite broad activist agendas on many fronts, the HIV-positive remain marginalized social constructors of HIV-disease. After that article was published, I proposed to the editor of the *Journal of Homosexuality* to collect and present a series of papers in which accounts of institutional control over the social construction of HIV-disease had dramatic impacts on the lives of HIV-positive people. Those papers are the essays in this volume.

THE DANGEROUS "FUNCTIONAL" VIEW OF ACTIVISM

To begin with, a rather "functional" view of activism has taken hold in some quarters of the broadly construed activist community. That is, an overarching conceptualization of "activism" on the part of many AIDS activists and academics has become almost "Poundian"—that is to say, much like the "functionalist" understanding of *law* developed by Roscoe Pound. Pound wrote: "I am content to think of law as a social institution to satisfy social wants" (Pound, 1921, pp. 91-93). Thus, Pound saw law as a form of holistic "social engineering" and espoused a model of law that was essentially "pluralistic"—meaning that he viewed the regulation of social conflict by law as an *effective* means of governing the fray of competing interests. According to Pound, on balance, law successfully serves the function of regulating opposing interests for the betterment of society.

In a similar vein, there is a tendency on the part of many AIDS activists and academics of late to view their activities as having successfully countered opposing interests in the popular presentation of the plight of the HIV-positive (Kinsella, 1989). In short, a "function" of the perceived "success" AIDS activists have had in the media is the faulty presumption that AIDS activists have conveyed the true meaning of HIV-disease through the media.

The suggestion that activists have failed to convey a construction of HIV-disease dominated by the HIV-positive did not fare well in some activist quarters. A criticism of our article partially read:

> it isn't hard to see how HIV/AIDS activists have achieved a
> presence and voice in the media . . . : Through a combination
> of homework and hell raising, ACT UP and other organiza-
> tions have forced their way into the news columns . . . by
> "acting up."

And, as another AIDS scholar put it upon reviewing the proposal
for this book:

> Gay and lesbian activists have led the fight against AIDS in
> this country, especially in the domain of public culture . . . Yes,
> gays are marginalized by mainstream America, but they are
> vocal and cannot be ignored.

The essays in this collection reject the assertion that activism has
been a highly effective remedy to HIV-positive voicelessness. This
collection of essays demonstrates that, in the battle for control over
the social construction of HIV-disease, AIDS activists *have well
been ignored and continue to be marginalized.*[4]
Certainly, AIDS activists have been highly aware of the fact that
they "must fight," must "ACT UP," to get their voices heard;
however, important transformations have taken place with regards
to the focus of activism that are instructive. As Michael Musheno
points out, today "neither ACT UP nor local networks of Injecting
Drug Users (IDUs) see the state as the focal point of their activities" (1994, p. 239). *The issue is not that activists have not been
vocal—it is that activists continue to be ignored in regards to the
social constructions of HIV disease, despite their vocality.*
This collection of writings offers numerous examples of institutional control and demonstrates that institutional structures, and not
activists, are "controlling the public meaning" of HIV-related
issues (a point also made by Watney, 1987, p. 22).

"Full-Blown": Winning Battles, Losing the War

A consequence of the lack of activist control over the social
construction of HIV-disease is the relative absence of HIV-positive
voices in public discourse about AIDS. When dominant social institutions put forward messages about HIV/AIDS, these messages

generally address concerns regarding how HIV relates to white, mainstream, heterosexual America (see chapter 2). This has been true from the beginning and it remains true today (Shilts, 1987; Kinsella, 1989). Why are social constructions so important to social policy? As Conrad and Schneider put it:

> Social policy may be characterized as an institutionalized definition of a problem and its solutions. There are many routes for developing social policy in a complex society, but, as John McKnight contends, "There is no greater power than the right to define the question" (reference omitted). The definition and the designation of the problem itself may be the key to the development of social policy. Problem definitions often take on a life of their own; they tend to resist change and become the accepted manner of defining reality. (1980, p. 17)[5]

Validation of the thesis of this book (the idea that to understand the sui generis nature of HIV-disease, one must first account for institutional power) is practically omnipresent: Simultaneous yet contradictory messages proliferate about HIV/AIDS—from accounts of outright "PLAGUE" to stories foreshadowing the much-prophesied, yet-still-admittedly-far-off "cure" or "vaccine" for HIV.[6] Additional messages conferring various legal, moral, and economic meanings on the epidemic proliferate as well. Perhaps all would agree that AIDS messages are in fact big business: The simultaneous culpability and risk faced by doctors, dentists, and nurses; the "innocence" of children, hemophiliacs, and transfusion patients; the implicit "guilt" of male homosexuals and IV drug users (AIDS initially being called "gay cancer" and "gay related immune deficiency"); the "successful" subsequent "curbing" of sex among gay men; the high costs of AIDS research and treatment as compared to breast cancer, heart disease, and prostate cancer; issues regarding drugs, promiscuity, and individual responsibility; HIV as *God's* method of population control; messages aplenty regarding potential routes of transmission (kisses, bites, blood transfusions, sex, drugs, trips to the dentist); and, most extraordinarily perhaps, the recent trend toward casting HIV/AIDS as "myth," a theme which played out heavily in the media in the wake of a book titled *The Myth of Heterosexual AIDS* (Fumento, 1990).

To say the least, current popular social constructions of HIV-disease are undeniably chaotic and often contradictory. What all of the above messages have in common, however, and what this volume takes as its starting point is that messages about HIV/AIDS are produced, negotiated, modified, and sustained through institutional mechanisms that serve mostly institutional interests. For example, as Ronald Bayer points out regarding Michael Fumento's book *The Myth of Heterosexual AIDS*: "[I]ts polemical thrust is directed at those who appealed for resources to meet the challenges of AIDS" in a context of shrinking budgets and budget deficits, and "it is in that light that Fumento's . . . [book] must be read" (1992, p. 208).

Thus, claims of various sorts regarding the relative threat of HIV are propagated by institutions that stand to gain or lose based on the extent to which their own version of AIDS "reality" is accepted or rejected. The most general of the assertions we wish to make here is that no mass-mediated message exists about HIV/AIDS that is free from institutionalized bias of some form–including this one.[7] Since AIDS messages are propagated by institutions *for institutional reasons* it is vitally important that we understand the workings of institutional power as we seek to reduce the level of marginalization continually endured by the HIV-positive. As Sander Gilman writes: "People have been stigmatized and destroyed as much by the *idea* of AIDS as by its reality. It is vital that we understand the social construction of AIDS, because it has directly affected the lives of so many" (1987, p. 88).

To begin our discussion, several "underpinning assertions" are presented below to guide the reader through the rest of the volume. These assertions form the academically grounded base upon which the rest of the volume stands. Each of these assertions is borne out somewhere in the following text.

UNDERPINNING ASSERTIONS

1. Competing HIV/AIDS "realities" exist–not all of which have been presented by the media nor are present in public discourse (Watney, 1987) [throughout; in particular, chapters 3, 4, 5].

2. The dominant social constructions of HIV/AIDS have been altered over time. These constructions convey only contextually limited and institutionally self-serving views of HIV/AIDS (Spector & Kitsuse, 1987; see also Schwartz & Leitko, 1977; Baker, 1986; Altman, 1986; Kinsella, 1989; Musheno et al., 1994) [chapters 3, 4, 5, 6].

3. The specific "reality" of a given HIV/AIDS message is that which various claims-makers have been permitted to define as such—these messages being further refined through association with specific institutional events and criteria (see Altheide, 1985; Ericson et al., 1989) [throughout].

4. Scientific/medical discourse is only one of several competing types of discourse operating in social constructions of HIV/AIDS as they are presented in the media. Other prominent discourses are "legal" and "public reaction" discourse and the discourse of government reports, each of which may contain elements of the others [especially chapters 2, 3, 6, 7].

5. Scientific/medical discourse is by far the dominant one in HIV/AIDS-specific messages published, and doctors and medical researchers are by far the dominant claims-makers present in mainstream HIV/AIDS-specific messages (see also Plumer, 1989, p. 25, for the "hegemony of medical science" in HIV-related discourse) [chapters 2, 3, 6, 7].

6. Persons with HIV/AIDS have little voice in AIDS-specific messages presented in the mainstream news media [chapter 2].

7. The voice of persons with HIV/AIDS is most prevalent in articles written to fill the "human interest" format of newspapers, where the particular story is focused on an individual's HIV-positive status and the plight associated with such status [chapter 2].

8. The hetero-centric bias of HIV/AIDS mainstream newspaper reporting, noted earlier by Baker (1986), Altman (1986), Shilts (1987), and Kinsella (1989), is further borne out here. Not only do people with HIV/AIDS have little voice in the mainstream press—but HIV/AIDS-specific messages are, on average, more than three times as likely to deal with *heterosexual* concerns than the concerns of homosexuals with HIV/AIDS [chapter 2].

SUMMARY OF CHAPTERS

To start the book off, the above-mentioned article, previously published in the *Journal of Homosexuality,* is presented in chapter 2. "Gatekeeping Through Media Format: Strategies of Voice for the HIV-Positive via Human Interest News Formats and Organizations" documents the lack of HIV-positive voice in mainstream news portrayals of HIV/AIDS and relates the paucity of citations from HIV-positive people to institutional routines, logic, and power. This chapter presents data from a content analysis of 535 major articles on the subject of HIV-disease and documents the sources cited as authorities in those articles. The chapter explores institutional dominion over popular discourse about HIV-disease and outlines how media-based interests have thwarted the voices of the HIV-positive in the context of the news media. The chapter concludes by making suggestions for future activism.

In chapter 3, "Truth and Deception in AIDS Information Brochures," the activist group National Council on HIV-Disease presents their research on state-government-level constructions of HIV-disease. This chapter documents state-governmental subversion of expansive constructions of HIV-disease (i.e., the notion that anyone can get HIV, for example, or that it is 99.9 percent fatal). Writes the National Council:

> While it is clear that governments frequently practice deception and secrecy with the justification that the public would become dangerously emotional and irrational if fully informed, there is no evidence that the public would, in fact, behave that way.

A ranking of state AIDS brochures for accuracy and totality of information is provided.

Chapters 4 and 5 deal more directly with social constructions and how they affect HIV/AIDS policy, first in a specific context (a county jail) and then (in chapter 5) in the broader framework of federal HIV/AIDS policy.

In chapter 4, "The Social Construction of Target Populations and the Transformation of Prison-Based AIDS Policy," Nancy Lynne Hogan utilizes an emergent model of constructionism (Schneider and Ingram's 1994 model of constructed "target populations") to explain alterations in policy and inmate status at a jail facility, the site of her previously published research on HIV/AIDS in correctional settings (Hogan, 1994). Here, Dr. Hogan tracks the development of officially generated constructions of HIV/AIDS with the evolutionary transformation of AIDS-based policy at the jail. As the social construction of HIV-disease was negotiated by inmates, guards, and jail administrators, policy at the jail changed as well. Hogan concludes by suggesting that power imbalances regarding inmates' inability to construct a version of HIV-disease that was nonthreatening, worked to ensure that transformations in jail-based AIDS policy were dominated by misinformation, fear, and repression. Consequently, officially generated AIDS policy reproduced constructions of HIV that were harmful to inmates and based on misinformation. Dr. Hogan concludes that, particularly with regard to HIV/AIDS education in correctional settings, HIV-positive inmates must be *allowed* to participate in the construction of correctional-based AIDS policy.

In chapter 5, Mark Donovan echoes themes presented in chapter 3 by the National Council for HIV-Disease, but writes about the consequences of social constructions and HIV-disease more broadly. In his chapter, "The Problem with Making AIDS Comfortable: Federal Policy Making and the Rhetoric of Innocence," Donovan discusses the extent to which policy makers at the federal level have been moved to action by symbolic representations of AIDS that are divorced from the reality of HIV-related suffering. AIDS-based policy has been governed by stereotypes promoted by institutionally driven, officially sanctioned and sanctified, versions of HIV-disease. As a result, Federal policy toward HIV-disease continues to distinguish between "deserving" and "undeserving" victims of HIV and, like the prison-based policies discussed in chapter 5, is best understood as representative of a "containment" logic designed to "narrow" and limit the scope of popular social constructions of HIV-disease (see also Musheno, Gregware, & Drass, 1991).

In chapter 6, "A Citizens' AIDS Task Force: Overcoming Obstacles," law professor Jane Aiken discusses her previous role as chair of a Western state's Governor's AIDS Task Force, outlining the political interests and battles fought over the political construction of AIDS and the interest-based struggles involved. This chapter speaks to the issue of institutional power in relation to activism in the context of the public health. Writes Professor Aiken: "This experience taught me that highly organized communities can affect policy making such that it offsets more institutionalized power. The only prerequisite is that institutionalized power must either perceive no threat from the policy or be looking the other way." Professor Aiken concludes that while her activist-dominated task force won on key issues in this case, their win was more a result of default by institutional power than the result of *displaced* institutional power. In the aftermath of activist victories, a systematic dismantling of activist-generated policies worked to reassert institutional power.

Finally, in chapter 7, "AIDS and the New Medical Gaze: Bio-Politics, AIDS, and Homosexuality," Professor Dion Dennis utilizes Foucauldian concepts to discuss the emergent "bio-politics" of HIV and homosexuality in the context of the United States–linking rights-oriented activists using genetic constructions for the basis of access to protected classes of rights to the possible damaging and constraining impacts of this strategy in the future lives of homosexuals. Specifically, Professor Dennis examines the ways in which biological categories traditionally have been used to justify exclusion rather than protection.

NOTES

1. As used in this text, "activism" is meant to include the broad spectrum of diverse activities commonly grouped under the umbrella term "activism." Activism includes: *Cultural Politics* (e.g., the AIDS quilt project), *Direct Action* taken in the context of New Social Movement activity (e.g., ACT UP), *Case Activism* (e.g., various AIDS Litigation Projects), *Self-Organization* (e.g., grass roots level self-help groups among Injecting Drug Users), and *Insider Alliances* within established political spheres (e.g., Harvey Milk) (see Gamson, 1989).

2. HIV-disease is currently the leading cause of death for Americans aged 25-44. The largest proportionate increases of late are reported among teens and young adults, mostly from *heterosexual* transmission. Through 1992, 47 percent of all reported AIDS cases were among blacks and Hispanics, while these two population groups represent only 21 percent of the total U.S. population. HIV-disease is currently among the top 10 causes of death for children 1 to 4 years old. Since 1 in 5 reported AIDS cases is diagnosed in the 20-29 age group and the

median incubation period between HIV infection and AIDS diagnosis is about 10 years, it is clear that many people who were diagnosed with AIDS in their 20s became infected as teenagers (CDC, 10/93). The World Health Organization's Global Programme on AIDS, as of January 1994, estimates that global HIV prevalence by the year 2000 will be between 30 and 40 million. With these increasing numbers, it is clear that the *social* impacts and justifications for exclusion related to HIV-disease will continue to intensify.

3. Some argue that portions of the activist community have been successful in disseminating messages about HIV/AIDS in popular culture; however, others argue that these messages have been co-opted and watered down by established institutional structures like Paramount Pictures and SONY, for example (Kramer, 1992). While large numbers of young people are dying and their friends, families, and loved ones are loudly vocal, the objective plight of the HIV-positive as a group remains grim and socially misunderstood: We can watch the movie *Philadelphia* and come away feeling conscientiously vindicated by the portrayal of a successful AIDS litigation battle, yet go home feeling still exceedingly fearful about HIV—*and never have it discussed in the dominant media that most HIV-positive people are unable to engage in legal battles, let alone win them, as portrayed in the movie* (Mason, 1993; Musheno, Gregware, & Drass, 1991). Pseudo-events promoted by institutional structures, like the American Music Awards and the Academy Awards, for example, will celebrate these productions as instances of successful AIDS activism.

4. Unlike Pound, criminologist Richard Quinney sees policy and law "not as a representation of compromise of diverse interests in society, but as the dominance of some interests over and at the expense of others" (Quinney, 1970, p. 34): "Some, because of their authority position in the interest structure, are able to have their interests represented in public policy" and others are not (ibid.). Quinney, then, would reject the "Poundian" conceptualization of activism mentioned above, because in a politically organized society it is never the case that segmented interests consensually bend to the will of other interests for the purposes of "social engineering"; rather, some groups win and some groups lose—social engineering be damned. Put another way, it is dangerous to assume that there is some large-scale ameliorative logic driving the skirmishes between activists and institutions. Cases are best understood on an individual basis. As Aiken and Musheno point out, occasionally "have-nots" do win in AIDS litigation—but this is generally not the case (1994; also Mason, 1993). (See also contributing author Mark Donovan's essay herein, "The Problem with Making AIDS Comfortable.") Today, institutionally governed fictions or dramas about HIV are beginning to displace the veritable truth about it: that HIV is the world's leading killer of young people, most of whom are voiceless and who lack the political, economic, and even physical strength to avail themselves of the small gains won by active segments on their behalf. (As noted earlier, the single largest proportional increase in the HIV-positive population of late, in the United States, has occurred among economically disenfranchised groups: minority women, African Americans of both genders, teenagers, and children.)

5. Thus, if "heterosexual AIDS" is a "myth," then why fund HIV-related research and treatment to a greater level than we do research in the area of heart disease and prostate cancer–two preeminent concerns among heterosexual men (Fumento, 1990)? Even though AIDS activists have been successful in promoting a construction of HIV as "something everyone can get," the fact remains that–officially at least–only so-called "target populations" need fear HIV. In other words, you only need fear HIV if you find yourself somehow fitting within officially defined parameters of inclusion. Two essays in this volume deal with "target populations" and HIV-disease.

6. Recent enthusiasm for combination drug treatments, which are still experimental (7/96), was muted by the comments of Dr. Michael O'Shaughnessy: "Even if the new treatments work as well as researchers hope, they are likely to be little use to most of the world's HIV-infected people, who cannot afford to pay $10,000 or $15,000 a year for them."

7. Support for this research came from the *Journal of Homosexuality* and from the Center for Research and Education in Sexuality at San Francisco State University. In many ways, the claims of the HIV-positive have been held captive to the superior mechanisms of message distribution that socially legitimized institutions, like the National Institutes of Health and the *New England Journal of Medicine,* have at their disposal (see chapter 2).

REFERENCES

Aiken, Jane, & Michael Musheno. (1994). Why have-nots win in the HIV litigation arena: socio-legal dynamics of extreme cases. *Law & Policy, 16*(3). (Introductory Essay).

Altheide, David. (1985). *Media power.* Beverly Hills, CA: Sage.

Altheide, David, & Robert Snow. (1979). *Media logic.* Beverly Hills, CA: Sage.

Altman, Dennis. (1986). *AIDS in the mind of America.* Garden City, NY: Anchor Press/Doubleday.

Baker, Andrea J. (1986). The portrayal of AIDS in the media: An analysis of articles in the *New York Times.* In D. Feldman & T. Johnson (Eds.), *The social dimensions of AIDS: Method and theory.* New York: Praeger.

Bayer, Ronald. (1989). *Private acts, public consequences.* New York: Free Press.

_____ . (1992). Entering the second decade: The politics of prevention, the politics of neglect. In Fee & Fox, *AIDS: The making of a chronic disease,* Berkeley, CA: University of California Press, pp. 207-226.

Cobb, Roger, & C.D. Elder. (1972). *Participation in American politics: The dynamics of agenda-building.* Boston, MA: Allyn and Bacon, Inc.

Cobb, Roger, Jennie Keith-Ross, & Marc Howard Ross. (1976). Agenda building as a comparative political process. *American Political Science Review, 70,* 126-138.

Collins, Patricia Hill. (1989). The social construction on invisibility. *Perspectives on Social Problems, 1,* 77-93.

Conrad, Peter, & Joseph Schneider. (1980). *Deviance & medicalization: From badness to sickness.* Toronto: The C.V. Mosby Company.

Ericson, Richard V., P.M. Baranek, & Janet B.L. Chan. (1989). *Negotiating control: A study of news sources.* Toronto: The C.V. Mosby Co.

Foucault, Michel. (1979). *Discipline & punish: The birth of the prison.* New York: Vantage Books.

Fumento, Michael. (1990). *The myth of heterosexual AIDS.* New York: Basic Books.

Gamson, Josh. (1989). Silence, death, and the invisible enemy: AIDS activism and social movement "newness," *Social Problems, 36,* 351-67.

Gilman, Sander. (1987). AIDS and syphilis: The iconography of disease. *October, 43,* 87-108.

Guba, Egon, & Yvonna Lincoln. (1989). *Fourth generation evaluation.* Beverly Hills, CA: Sage.

Hallett, Michael A. (1994). Why we fail at crime control. In *Declaring peace on crime,* Robert Elias, Special Issues Editor, *Peace Review, 6*(2), 177-182.

Hallett, Michael A., & David Cannella. (1994). Gatekeeping through media format: Media strategies for the HIV-positive. *Journal of Homosexuality, 26*(4), 111-137.

Hallett, Michael A., & Robert Rogers. (1994). The push for truth in sentencing: Evaluating competing stakeholder constructions. The case for contextual constructionism in evaluation research. *Evaluation & Program Planning, 17* (2), 187-196.

Hogan, Nancy Lynne. (1994). HIV education for inmates: Uncovering strategies for program selection. *The Prison Journal, 74*(2), 220-243.

Keniston, Kenneth. (1990). Introduction to the issue. In Stephen R. Graubard (Ed.), *Living with AIDS.* Cambridge, MA: The MIT Press.

Kinsella, James. (1989). *Covering the plague: AIDS and the American media.* Brunswick, NJ: Rutgers University Press.

Kitzinger, Jenny. (1990). Audience understandings of AIDS media messages: A discussion of methods. *Sociology of Health and Illness, 12* (3), 319-335.

Kramer, Larry. (1992). Kramer vs. Kramer. *Vanity Fair,* October, p. 228.

Mason, Belinda Ann. (1993). A seat on the merry go round: A consumer's view. In *AIDS law today: A new guide for the public.* Scott Burris et al. (Eds.). New Haven: Yale.

Miller, Leslie. (1993). Claimsmaking from the underside: Marginalization and social problems analysis. In Miller, Gale, & James Holstein, *Perspectives on social problems.* New York: JAI Press, 1989. Vol. 1, pp. 1-16.

Musheno, Michael C. (1994). Introductory essay. Socio-legal dynamics of AIDS: Constructing identities, protecting boundaries amidst crisis. In Michael Musheno (Ed.), "Special Issue on the Socio-Legal Dynamics of AIDS," *Law & Policy, 16*(3).

Musheno, Michael C., Peter Gregware, & Kriss Drass. (1991). Court management of AIDS disputes: A sociolegal analysis. *Law & Social Inquiry, 16,* 737-74.

Palumbo, Dennis J., & Michael A. Hallett. (1992). "Conflict versus consensus models in policy evaluation and implementation." *Evaluation and Program Planning, 16*, 1-13.

Palumbo, Dennis J., Michael C. Musheno, & Michael A. Hallett. (1994). The political construction of criminal justice alternatives: Alternatives to incarceration and alternative dispute resolution. *Evaluation & Program Planning, Special Edition: Emergent Trends in Evaluation Research.*

Plumer, Kenneth. (1989). Organizing AIDS. In Peter Aggleton & Hilary Homans (Eds.), *Social aspects of AIDS.* New York: The Falmer Press.

Pound, Roscoe. (1921). *The spirit of the common law.* Boston, MA: Marshall Jones.

Quinney, Richard. (1970). *The social reality of crime.* Boston, MA: Little Brown.

Schwartz, J.P., & Thomas Leitko. (1977). The rise of social problems: Newspapers as thermometers. In Mauss, Armaund L., & Julie Camile, *This land of promises.* Philadelphia, PA: Lippencott, pp. 427-436.

Shilts, Randy. (1987). *And the band played on: Politics, people, and the AIDS epidemic.* New York: St. Martin's Press.

Sontag, Susan. (1989). *AIDS and its metaphors.* New York: Doubleday.

Spector, Malcolm, & John I. Kitsuse. (1987). *Constructing social problems.* Menlo Park, CA: Cummings.

Stipp, Horst, & Dennis Kerr. (1989). Determinants of public opinion about AIDS. *Public Opinion Quarterly, 53*, 98-106.

Thomas, George M., John W. Meyer, Francisco O. Ramirez, & John Boli. (1987). *Institutional structure: Constituting state, society, and the individual.* Beverly Hills, CA: Sage Publications.

Watney, Simon. (1989). The subject of AIDS. In Peter Aggleton, Graham Hart, & Peter Davies (Eds.), *AIDS: Social representations, social practices.* New York: Falmer Press.

_____ . (1987). *Policing desire: Pornography, AIDS, and the media.* London: Comedia, Methuen & Co. Ltd.

Gatekeeping Through Media Format: Strategies of Voice for the HIV-Positive via Human Interest News Formats and Organizations

Michael A. Hallett, PhD

Middle Tennessee State University

David Cannella, BS

Arizona State University

SUMMARY. This research examines the extent to which HIV-positive voices are marginalized in the mainstream versus the "alternative" press. The central claim of this research is that news media for-

Michael A. Hallett is Assistant Professor of Criminal Justice Administration at Middle Tennessee State University. David Cannella is the Medical Writer for the *Arizona Republic*. Special thanks to Michael Musheno.

This research was supported in part by a grant from the Arizona State University Graduate College Research and Development Program, grant # CIR-D582, and by a National Science Foundation grant, Law and Social Science Program, # SES-8908456. Additional thanks is due the editorial and reportorial staffs of the *Arizona Republic* and the Phoenix *New Times*, without whose enthusiastic assistance this project would not have been possible.

Correspondence may be addressed: Department of Criminal Justice Administration, Middle Tennessee State University, Murfreesboro, TN 37132.

This article is reprinted from *Journal of Homosexuality,* Volume 26, Number 4, 1994.

[Haworth co-indexing entry note]: "Gatekeeping Through Media Format: Strategies of Voice for the HIV-Positive via Human Interest News Formats and Organizations." Hallett, Michael A., and David Cannella. Co-published simultaneously in *Journal of Homosexuality* (The Haworth Press, Inc.) Vol. 32, No. 3/4, 1997, pp. 17-36; and: *Activism and Marginalization in the AIDS Crisis* (ed: Michael A. Hallett) The Haworth Press, Inc., 1997, pp. 17-36; and: *Activism and Marginalization in the AIDS Crisis* (ed: Michael A. Hallett) Harrington Park Press, an imprint of The Haworth Press, Inc., 1997, pp. 17-36. Single or multiple copies of this article are available for a fee from The Haworth Document Delivery Service [1-800-342-9678, 9:00 a.m. - 5:00 p.m. (EST). E-mail address: get info@haworth.com].

mat considerations, constructed around what has come to be called "media logic," leave persons who are HIV-positive with comparatively little voice in the mainstream press. By utilizing techniques of content analysis, the research examines 535 major HIV/AIDS-specific stories published in two oppositional papers toward an assessment of the level of HIV-positive voice in each outlet. While arguments of "homophobia" have been previously used to explain bias in mainstream HIV/AIDS-coverage, this article asserts that "heterocentric" bias is, in fact, embedded in the routinized practices of mainstream "news production." The article concludes by suggesting that successful future HIV/AIDS-activism demands a recognition of "media logic" and an adoption of its tactics. *[Article copies available for a fee from The Haworth Document Delivery Service: 1-800-342-9678. E-mail address: getinfo@haworth.com]*

The most effective form of resistance to the hegemonic force of the dominant media is to speak for oneself. At one level this means attempting to be included in the category of recognized positions and groupings acknowledged by the mass media. Achieving this degree of legitimation is not a negligible accomplishment, and it is not to be despised or rejected as an important minority goal.

Larry Gross

Documenting the mainstream news media's hetero-centric bias with regards to its HIV/AIDS-news coverage has been the dominant task of HIV/AIDS-media research to this point (Baker, 1986; Altman, 1986; Albert, 1986; Stipp & Kerr, 1989; Kinsella, 1989; Watney, 1987).[1] It is clear from this research that the mainstream news media paid little attention to HIV/AIDS until fears of transmission to the dominant culture were reaffirmed by medical testimony (Altman, 1986; Baker, 1986; Kinsella, 1989). That is, as long as HIV/AIDS transmission remained conceptually confined to the homosexual and IV drug-using communities, the mainstream news media paid it little attention (Kinsella, 1989; Baker, 1986; Altman, 1986).[2]

This article extends earlier HIV/AIDS-media studies by utilizing a content analysis of two opposing Arizona newspapers, the *Arizona Republic* and the Phoenix *New Times*, a Phoenix-based weekly "alternative magazine,"[3] toward an analysis of the levels of voice of the HIV-positive.[4] This research examines over 535 major HIV/AIDS-specific articles appearing over a five-year period, from 1986 to 1990–including every major HIV/AIDS article published in each outlet during those years.[5]

The central claim of this research is that news media format strictures, constructed around what has come to be called "media-logic," leave persons who are HIV-positive with comparatively little voice in the mainstream press. Specifically, the hetero-centric bias of HIV/AIDS-news coverage documented by earlier scholars, which ignored the disenfranchised voices of HIV-positive gays and IV drug users, *has now altered in form* as HIV/AIDS has spread through the population: While today hardly a day goes by without an HIV/AIDS-specific article somewhere in the pages of a newspaper, the *systematic* exclusion of HIV-positive voices from HIV/AIDS-specific news media discourse continues.

By specifically tracking the level of HIV-positive voice in two newspapers of different operational formats, we illustrate that the patterned format considerations of news organizations virtually determine whose opinion gets published. These differences have profound implications for the "social construction" of HIV/AIDS as well as for the formulation of social policy and concepts of social responsibility.

HIV/AIDS-scholar Simon Watney has suggested that "the precise mechanisms of how gay men and lesbians are regarded in and by this industry (the media) remains an important question and one which has been significantly overlooked" (Watney, 1987a). The HIV/AIDS-news media relationship must be reassessed and further scrutinized in terms of its biased HIV/AIDS reporting. We argue here that the complex nature and depth of news media hetero-centrism reveals itself in very specific ways with regards to HIV/AIDS-"news" reporting and illustrate these here.

HIV/AIDS AND THE AMERICAN MEDIA: REVIEW OF THE LITERATURE

To define AIDS as "God's judgement on a society that does not live by the rules," as does Rev. Jerry Falwell, directs us toward blame, penitence, and moral reform as the only effective responses to this affliction. To see AIDS as an entirely biomedical problem deflects us from promoting behavioral changes that could limit its transmission. To view it as a problem likely to be solved in the near future undermines the resolve needed to live with AIDS for decades and generations. We must therefore weigh the competing social constructions of AIDS against what we know about this condition and against whether they promote policies that can reduce the damage HIV causes. (Keniston, 1990)

"AIDS has forced reporters to acknowledge that their treatment of the news, far from being objective, is often shaped by their personal prejudices and their assumptions about their audience" writes James Kinsella in *Covering the Plague: AIDS and the American Media* (1989, p. 1). The media has been "the primary vehicle for both formal and informal messages about AIDS" and "for the population at large, those with no direct contact with AIDS or its sufferers, the awareness of the disease is media related" (Kitzinger, 1990, p. 319).

The "Gay Disease"

HIV/AIDS's American origin as a predominantly "gay disease," initially being labeled "Gay-Related Immune Deficiency" or "GRID" (also variously cited as Gay-Related Infectious Disease) by the medical community, has had a significant impact on how Americans perceive and react to the phenomenon generally (Stipp & Kerr, 1989; Thomas, 1989; Watney, 1988, 1989).[6] In fact, "until 1983, articles on HIV/AIDS could be located under the listing of "Homosexuality" in the *Times Index* and also in *The Reader's Guide to Periodical Literature*" (Baker, 1986, p. 243). In sum, as Dennis Altman writes: "The fact that the first reported cases were exclusively among gay men was to affect the whole future (American) conceptualization of AIDS" (1986, p. 33).

Furthermore, the government's initial lack of attention to the problems of HIV/AIDS had a tremendous impact on how the media chose to cover the subject: "Without the government taking AIDS seriously, and without individual journalists being seized by the seriousness of the epidemic, the disease became a kind of curio" (Kinsella, 1989, p. 3; Shilts, 1987, p. 121). It has also been noted that "to explain AIDS transmission, words like 'semen' and 'penis' and 'vagina' are absolutely essential. Unfortunately, in the first years of the epidemic, they were strictly avoided" and the subject ignored (Kinsella, 1989, p. 3).[7]

Thus, HIV/AIDS's early association with homosexuality–and our society's correspondent lack of attention to the problems of homosexuals–worked to inhibit mainstream news media presentation of the issues–not to mention (and they didn't) the terms with which discussions of HIV/AIDS must be associated (e.g., "penis," "anus," "semen," etc.). But it is insufficient to assume that homophobia and the need for unprecedented types of language can fully explain the persistent lack of HIV-positive voice in HIV/AIDS-news media discourse. Some deeper, more structural, explanation is warranted.

THEORETICAL BASE: MEDIA LOGIC

In the process of "news construction," news organizations adopt a certain operational logic ("media logic") which impacts heavily upon the levels and types of coverage a given issue or group receives (see Altheide & Snow, 1991). News organizations use this logic to manage the numerous competing claims to "news-worthiness" they confront daily. "Media logic" facilitates an *ordering* of these claims and acts as a filter through which a sifting of "news-worthy" information takes place–expediting the construction of raw information into a presentable "news" form.[8] In other words, as "news" is produced, a kind of governing takes place over the production of information ranked as "news."

The Privileging of Organizational Sources

In the process of producing a day's "news," news organizations routinely turn to social agencies or institutions for their information–so much so that "news" production has become limited by "an over reliance on selected people as knowledge resources"– especially, "key spokesperson for bureaucratic organizations"

(Ericson, Baranek, & Chan, 1989, p. 1; Altheide & Snow, 1979, 1991; Altheide, 1976). Thus, the question for the thinking reader/ viewer becomes: "What were we *told* was the news today and why?" rather than simply: "What was the news today?"

This privileging of organizational sources by the news media is a product of the formula used to "produce" news and to continually supply product—that is, "news" text. In short, from the perspective of the news organization, "media logic" is a necessary part of the division of labor: In order to effectively "report on" how a community is responding to all of its various "problems," a logical, standardized response has become to first turn to society's organizations and to report from these sources what is being (or ought to be) done.

The problem with this approach is that it operationalizes a series of media-based assumptions that facilitate a *privileging* of information that comes from only (certain) organizations. In other words, all organizations are not treated equally in the news production hierarchy (Ericson et al., 1989). A built-in bias exists that presupposes that information from an organization like the Centers for Disease Control (CDC), for example, is more reliable and valid than information from a group like ACT UP—because, after all, CDC employs certain "scientifically valid" procedures which lend legitimacy to the news organization itself. This legitimacy allows the news organization to play off the information as "responsible" journalism. This, of course, is not to mention the millions of dollars in research money already invested in legitimizing CDC generally (see also Conrad & Schneider, 1980). In sum, organizational citations are viewed as more socially responsible and "safe" journalism for the news organization.

Shaping Reality

The theoretical rudiments of "media logic" may be found in the scholarship of symbolic interactionist Georg Simmel, who argued that "form is a process through which reality is rendered intelligible. Form is not structure per se, but a processual *framework through which social action occurs*" (Altheide & Snow, 1991, p. 12, emphasis added). That is to say, there is a rather complex interface between the content of a news message as delivered from its source and the news organization's presentation of that information. Before a message is delivered through print or over the air, *a process of "negotiation" takes place* between the source of "news" and the news organization itself (Ericson et al., 1989). As media scholar Richard Ericson has written: "Through journalists, sources seek to construct an organizational order that is partial: partial to their own interests, and offering only a partial version of social order" (Ericson et al., 1989, p. 16).

Thus, "all organizations [seek to] control knowledge of their activity in order to sustain the view publicly that they are operating with procedural regularity, and are therefore accountable" (Ericson et al., 1989, p. 92). In fact, sources actively solicit reporters with organizational awards and "press kits" which help them write their stories from that organization's perspective (Ericson et al., 1989, pp. 1-33).[9] As one reporter told us: "What really influences who gets quoted in the news, is who has managed to get themselves into the reporter's Rolodex."

It is important to note, therefore, that this "media" logic has not gone unnoticed by societal organizations themselves—who now have "public relations officers" and advertising firms working to assemble information in *media-ready* packages—helping to ensure the airing and/or publication of their organization-centered information (e.g., press kits). As Richard Ericson writes:

> In the contemporary knowledge society news represents *who* are the authorized knowers and *what* are their authoritative versions of reality. As such, it is every person's daily barometer of "the knowledge structure of society." It offers a perpetual articulation of how society is socially stratified in terms of possession of knowledge [and] . . . At the same time that it informs about who are the authorized knowers, it suggests, by relegation to a minor role and by omission, who is excluded from having a say in important matters. (Ericson et al., 1989, pp. 3-4)

MEDIA LOGIC AND FORMATS OF CONTROL: HETERO-CENTRISM IN ACTION

On November 14, 1990, the front page of the *New York Times* read: "NEWS OF ADVANCE IN AIDS TREATMENT DELAYED 5 MONTHS, Advocates are angered." The ensuing article explained that medical scientists had discovered that treatment with steroid hormones can halve the death rate from the pneumonia that is the leading killer of people with AIDS. But it was five months before the government agency that convened the experts notified doctors who treat AIDS patients of the finding. (*New York Times,* 11/14/90, A-1)

The reason given by the National Institute of Allergy and Infectious Diseases about why the findings had not been made public immediately is that:

The papers had not yet been accepted at a prestigious medical journal, and the authors feared that an announcement of the findings would jeopardize their publication. (*New York Times,* 11/14/90, A-1)

Of the five medical trials done involving the steroid treatment, one study had results so effective that the experiment was terminated after just 23 patients were enrolled "because the group that received the steroids did so much better," reported the *Times.*

A doctor involved in the research finally convinced editors of the journal in question, the *New England Journal of Medicine,* to let the findings out before publication in the journal—but succeeded only after the journal had secured publication slots for two of the five studies involved. Said the doctor: "It is clear that there are people whose lives may be saved if their doctors knew about the steroids" (*NYT,* 11/14/90, A-1).

The important point, obviously, is that the institute had chosen not to notify the press of the steroid recommendation because the *New England Journal of Medicine,* like other leading medical journals, has a policy against publishing studies that have been previously described in the press. *Thus, institutional acceptance and response defined "success" in this case—and not the overwhelming results of the data.* The successful application of steroids to patients who could have used them was *not* the defining moment of the study—publication of the results was.

Everyone's Interest but the HIV-Positive

Thus, we have a clear HIV/AIDS-specific example of media logic driving organizational (and societal) responses to a social problem: Here, the "institutional agenda" defined success for researchers and patients and doctors. This is the important way in which media logic generally has been "hetero-centric" and impacted upon the HIV/AIDS issue: the considerations of people with HIV/AIDS have been secondary to the concerns of the social institutions dealing with the problem—be it the medical community or the news media. In this case, media logic physically controlled the parameters of the entire situation: "For months the researchers struggled to find a way to draft a statement that would not jeopardize their chances of publication and that correctly reflected their analysis of the data," reported the *Times* (*NYT,* 11/14/90, A-1). The authors "could not agree on the wording of a statement" that would not jeopardize their own publications and chose to acquiesce (*NYT,* 11/14/91, A-1).

"The Inglefinger Rule"

The publication policy in question at the *NEJM* is called the "Inglefinger Rule," titled after the late editor of the journal, Dr. Franz Inglefinger, and it has come under criticism before:

> Although the written version of the policy seems innocuous enough, its application in practice appears to stifle communication among members of the research community. Colleagues are reluctant to talk about their work even informally lest they jeopardize their chances of having their work published in a journal that is for many of them the key to professional advancement. . . . It is my thesis that the Inglefinger Rule exists . . . to enhance the economic position of the journal. (Dr. E. Reinhardt, Princeton University, *NYT,* 2/10/88, A-30)

In turn, the *New England Journal of Medicine*'s justification for enforcing the Inglefinger Rule is that "doctors cannot give sound advice on the basis of a broadcast or a newspaper story. Therefore, the *Journal* should be in the hands of its medical subscribers before the press alerts their patients" (*NYT,* 2/10/88, A-30).

Arguments made by doctors against the rule include the lengthy review process of the *Journal* as well as the fact that most of the research reported in the *Journal* is supported by tax-generated monies. Furthermore, while there are over 600,000 practicing physicians in the United States, only some 185,000 subscribe to the journal (*Chicago Tribune*, 2/17/88, A-17). It thus makes more sense to release the findings early to the press, in order to help spread the word to the majority of doctors across the country who do *not* subscribe to the *Journal*, so that they may then judge for themselves whether they need to seek out the findings in the *New England Journal of Medicine* and go about utilizing information with their dying patients. It was the opinion of the researchers themselves in this case that news of the steroid treatment would have saved the lives of AIDS patients. Doctors, hearing about the findings could have judged for themselves whether they knew enough to immediately begin treating dying patients with the appropriate steroids.

Thus, the media logic of the *New England Journal of Medicine* is quite apparent: By withholding information under the rhetoric of "meticulous examination of findings" and the "medical autonomy of doctors," the *New England Journal of Medicine* was able to successfully control the flow of information which is its primary source of capital: breakthrough research findings in the medical sciences. In sum, institutional interests were put above the interests of individual patients.

ASSERTIONS MADE BASED ON THE COLLECTED DATA

The following assertions are made based on the data collected for this research:

1. Institutional affiliation has a direct bearing on the level and type of coverage HIV/AIDS receives in the mainstream news media. "While individuals without organizational affiliation are cited—especially in designated places such as letters-to-the-editor columns, or for specific news purposes such as to inspire 'fear and loathing' over a tragic event in a news story—they are a small minority statistically" (Ericson et al., 1989, p. 1).

2. Scientific/medical discourse is only one of several competing types of discourse operating in social constructions of HIV/AIDS as they are presented in the news media. (Other promi-

nent discourses are "legal" and "public reaction" discourse and the discourse of government reports, each of which may contain elements of the others.)

3. Medical discourse is by far the dominant one in HIV/AIDS-specific news articles published, and doctors and medical researchers are by far the dominant claims-makers present in the HIV/AIDS-specific articles examined, resulting in the so-called "hegemony of medical discourse" in HIV/AIDS reporting (see Plumer, 1988, p. 25; Conrad & Schneider, 1980, p. 249). ("Medical definitions have a high likelihood for dominance and hegemony; they are often taken as the last scientific word. The language of medical experts increases mystification and decreases the accessibility of public debate" [Conrad & Schneider, 1980, p. 249].)

4. Persons with HIV/AIDS have little voice in HIV/AIDS-specific articles presented in the news media, except where they are affiliated with some organization or where they fill the "human interest" news format. Here the particular story is focused on an individual's HIV-positive status and the plight associated with such status.

FINDINGS

The Voice of People with HIV/AIDS

Percentage of HIV/AIDS-Specific Stories
Citing HIV-Positive

	86	87	88	89	90
in *Arizona Republic*	4	15	21	26	25
in *Phoenix New Times*	100	83	92	—	100

As shown above, the voice of people with HIV/AIDS has increased steadily in the *Republic* since 1986. The *Republic,* however, only published an average of about 20 percent of HIV/AIDS-specific articles that cited HIV-positive sources over the five-year period.

In the *New Times,* however, for the period examined, an average of 75 percent of the total HIV/AIDS-specific articles published cited people with HIV/AIDS.[10] This made people with HIV/AIDS the most frequently cited source in *New Times* HIV/AIDS-specific coverage and illustrates the marked difference in operational format of the two papers. The implication is that the mainstream press has not yet decided to seek out HIV-positive sources for their HIV/AIDS coverage. What this means, as Simon Watney aptly points out, is that HIV-negative people are "controlling the public meaning" of an illness they don't have (1987a, p. 22).

Percentage of HIV/AIDS-Specific Stories
Citing Organizational Sources

	86	87	88	89	90
in *Arizona Republic*	95	97	92	94	92
in *Phoenix New Times*	40	52	43	–	39

The impact of media logic on HIV/AIDS-news reporting is illustrated by the above findings: Where dominant institutionalized sources such as the Centers for Disease Control, local public health agencies, and various institutionally backed medical research agencies were concerned–there was substantial presence of voice. Over 90% of all *Arizona Republic* HIV/AIDS-specific stories over the five-year research period cited organizational sources. Where largely disenfranchised HIV-positive individuals were concerned, however–particularly HIV-positive homosexuals, HIV-positive women, and HIV-positive inmates–they had virtually no voice in the mainstream Arizona newspaper. What needs to happen is that media logic must somehow incorporate the notion that people with HIV/AIDS are valid sources for HIV/AIDS-specific information.

Human Interest: The HIV-Positive Format

Percentage of HIV/AIDS-Specific Stories
Which Were Human Interest

	86	87	88	89	90
in *Arizona Republic*	10	10	18	11	13
in *Phoenix New Times*	100	40	48	–	100

Due to the operational dictates of media logic, the primary location of HIV-positive voice in both newspapers examined was in the "human interest" format. Human interest stories portray HIV/AIDS patients or doctors as either suffering or heroic and create attitudes of sympathy or horror in the reader. The primary trait of the human interest story is that it is written with an individual being the primary "source," rather than a bureaucratic organization. This characterization does not extend to all persons who are HIV-positive, however: HIV-positive children often have the backing of an institution like a hospital or charity and often receive amplified voice via these organizational news sources.

Levels of Coverage

Number of Major HIV/AIDS Stories

	86	87	88	89	90
in *Arizona Republic*	51	163	135	83	85
in *Phoenix New Times*	1	9	6	—	1

As shown above, levels of HIV/AIDS coverage peaked in 1987 for the *Arizona Republic* and hit a simultaneous high in that year for the *New Times*. The *Republic* published 163 major HIV/AIDS-specific articles in 1987 and the *New Times* published 9 major HIV/AIDS-specific stories. The important point gleaned from this data is that while the smaller paper did not have the resources to publish as many HIV/AIDS-specific stories as the *Republic*, the presence of voice of the HIV-positive was much higher in the smaller paper.

The simultaneous coverage peak in 1987 is due to the so-called "second wave" of the AIDS epidemic, during which Hispanic and black minorities were being found HIV-positive in record numbers. "From late 1986 on, the figures on those coming down with the disease showed that AIDS was claiming two and three times as many victims, proportionately, among those two minority groups than among whites" (Kinsella, 1989, p. 248). In addition, it was in October, 1986, that "the CDC warned public health officials that until an effective therapy or vaccine is available, prevention of HIV infection depends on education and behavioral modification of persons at increased risk" (Kinsella, 1990, p. 246). Numerous stories dealt with these two issues during 1987 and 1988.

Dominant "Types" of HIV/AIDS-Specific Coverage

Arizona Republic

1986	Medical/Scientific Update	59 %
1987	Public Reaction	50 %
1988	Public Reaction	42 %
1989	Medical/Scientific Update	31 %
1990	Medical/Scientific Update	39 %

Phoenix *New Times*

1986	Human Interest	100 %
1987	Human Interest	40 %
1988	Human Interest	48 %
1989	none	—
1990	Human Interest	100 %

As shown above, the dominant "type" of HIV/AIDS-specific article published in the *Republic* was not uniform over the period examined.[11] In 1986, the dominant "type" HIV/AIDS-specific article published in the *Republic* was "medical/scientific update."[12] For the next two years, however, 1987 and 1988, the dominant "type" of HIV/AIDS-specific article appearing in the *Republic* was "public reaction" articles focusing on public reactions to HIV/AIDS in their communities.[13] "Public reaction" stories, however, still relied heavily on medical/scientific testimony in their discourse.

HIV/AIDS-specific articles in the *New Times* tended to be longer in length than those in the *Republic,* in part due to the nature of the publication itself and in part due to the "type" of articles published there: 57.6 percent of all *New Times* HIV/AIDS-specific articles published were "human interest" stories—and therefore the prevalence of HIV-positive voice was generally higher and more consistent in the *Phoenix New Times*–the "alternative" newspaper–than in the "paper of historical record," the *Republic*. Thus, persons with HIV/AIDS had a stronger voice in the *New Times* than did the "medical/scientific" community and also had a stronger voice relative to all other voices–but in the broader scheme of media coverage in Arizona, the HIV-positive got much less.

INTERVIEWS: BLAMING THE VICTIM

According to editors and reporters at the *Arizona Republic,* what has kept the voice of the HIV-positive out of mainstream press, at least in the first half of the AIDS decade, was largely the HIV-positive themselves. In an interesting case of "blaming the victim," the news editor at the *Republic* from 1985 to 1991, said the HIV-positive "had no voice because they didn't put one forward."

The news editor is charged with selecting stories from the wire services that would run in the newspaper, as well as having an active role in deciding the play local stories on AIDS received. In the early to mid 1980s, the HIV-positive and those with full-blown AIDS were not speaking out, and therefore were neither heard by nor portrayed in the media: "They weren't speaking at public hearings, or giving speeches or making their voices known, and that is reflected in media coverage," said the editor.

This lack of voice was actually a product of fear of being identified publicly, of losing one's employment, of being branded a "queer" or "fag," according to three HIV-positive men we interviewed for this research. "Unlike San Francisco or New York," they explained, "here in Phoenix there was little local support for the HIV-positive and hardly no existing social network to which someone with HIV could turn."

The editor admitted, however, that "early on, I don't think anyone understood the geometric impact AIDS would have on society"–the point of this being that reporters, especially those in cities not heavily impacted by AIDS, did not seek out the HIV-positive because they did not think the story had (heterosexual) societal impact (see also Kinsella, 1989). In short, homosexuals dying of HIV/AIDS were not of mainstream news interest.

CONCLUSION

Strategies of Voice for the HIV-Positive: On the Efficacy of Activism

The workings of "media logic" and the processes of "news" production currently prescribe that news sources either be affiliated with large, socially legitimized institutions or that they supply stories which can be easily used by news organizations themselves. The dominant sources found in the articles examined for this research were invariably institutionally affiliated–resulting in an absence of voice for the disenfranchised HIV-positive–and a proliferation of voice for dominant cultural institutions.

While it would seem that truly "objective reporting" would focus on the problem where the problem still is–largely in the homosexual community–this has not happened. The hetero-centric bias documented by earlier scholars has yet to be overcome–and has even become further entrenched as HIV/AIDS spreads through the heterosexual population: the mainstream press now routinely relies on established dominant-culture organizations–like the CDC and the *New England Journal of Medicine*–for its HIV/AIDS information.

The recognizable problem, then, is that the process of news production itself works against the inclusion of voices that are disenfranchised–that is, not organizationally affiliated. The HIV-positive, then, continue to have little voice in the mainstream press because they are not affiliated with dominant cultural organizations. By casting the personal testimony of the HIV-positive consistently into the "human interest" format, information from the HIV-positive is not routinely worked into stories about HIV/AIDS–where dominant social institutions have spoken. What this means, as Simon Watney aptly points out, is that HIV-negative people are "controlling the public meaning" of an illness they don't have (1987a, p. 22).

Thus, the HIV-positive are left with few options. The former medical writer at the *Arizona Republic* told us that the HIV-positive are "going to have to play the game and serve up human interest stories" if they want their voice in the press. The problem with this is that publicly sharing views and experiences, even anonymously, is not something that many HIV-positive are willing to do: Incidents of violence, loss of employment, housing, insurance, and even friendships work to prevent such outspokenness in the majority of American cities. (Hetero-centrism in the media is just one form of discrimination endured by the HIV-positive.)

So, what should be done? The initial response is that we need to continue to "ACT UP." This argument suggests that by becoming a loud(er) voice of protest and engaging in civil disobedience, the media will have no choice but to hear–and print–what we have to say. Unfortunately, this is not what has happened. The mainstream press has *continued* to ignore the voices of the HIV-positive in its HIV/AIDS-specific "news"–despite the fact that activism has reached new heights in recent years (Altman, 1986). Many of the stories examined for this research came off of the national wire–many from San Francisco and New York, where the HIV-positive are comparatively quite active–and yet organizational sources continued to dominate the "news."

Thus, the problem is not one simply of activism, but one of complex relationships of power and influence and social legitimacy in the workings of "media logic." What is going on here is that the mainstream media is gatekeeping through media format: they are deciding who is "legitimate" in the "news"/knowledge hierarchy. The HIV-positive are excluded from big stories because they are not (yet) viewed as legitimate "news" sources. Policies like the *NEJM*'s "Inglefinger Rule" illustrate how entrenched, complex, and political institutional interests are in driving the coverage of HIV/AIDS–and highlight just how far we still have to go in terms of activism. The trick is to get into print.

In short, we need *new forms* of activism–forms of activism that *incorporate* "media logic" into their agendas. For example, Reuters news organization recently challenged the Inglefinger Rule when the *New England Journal of Medicine* tried to suppress findings of a Heart-Aspirin study. The *New England Journal of Medicine* threatened an "embargo" of Reuters, cutting off all *NEJM* contact with Reuters. A "news embargo" from a major source of societal "news" can be extremely damaging for a news organization, since being the "first" and "most complete" "news" is the mandate of many news organizations.

This kind of media-based orchestration needs to be challenged on the grounds that media control of important social information is harmful to all. We need to keep ourselves informed of these developments and, more importantly, on a micro level, the HIV-positive need to get their voice into the mainstream press. Literally getting your name into the address book of the health reporter at the nearest mainstream newspaper and offering to talk with reporters—with assurances of anonymity, if desired—is one solid place to start. Journalists are the "gatekeepers" of popular opinion: activists must devise ways to get through that gate. An awareness and *adoption* of "media logic," then, is going to be the key to successful activism in the future.

NOTES

1. The acronym "HIV/AIDS" indicates all persons who are HIV-positive and living with the full spectrum of life-threatening conditions that often accompany HIV-infection including the stigma associated with finding one's self HIV-positive. As Sander Gilman writes: "People have been affected as much by the *idea* of AIDS as by its reality" (1987, p. 88).

2. "Hetero-centric" is used throughout this article to connote journalistic activity undertaken strictly from the standpoint of heterosexual society.

3. The *Arizona Republic* and the *New Times* have fundamentally different operational formats. The *New Times* does not subscribe to the wire services nor cover major national or world events. The byline of the *New Times* is "Taking a Stand on the Issues" and "alternative magazine" are the words used by the HIV/ AIDS reporter of the *New Times* to describe that publication. The *Arizona Republic,* on the other hand, is the "paper of historical record" for Arizona, being the single largest daily metropolitan newspaper in Arizona, subscribing to the wire services and relaying world, national, and local stories "in an objective fashion."

4. "Level of voice" indicates the extent to which the voices of HIV-positive persons are present within a news article, in the form of quoted citations within the news text.

5. From the *Arizona Republic* all "medium" and "long" HIV/AIDS-specific articles were examined. Short blurbs about AIDS benefits, study reports, etc. were not examined. The characterizations "medium" and "long" are those of the *Arizona Republic,* "medium" articles being 70 lines or longer, and "long" articles consisting of 120 lines or more. All HIV/AIDS-specific articles published in the *New Times* over the five-year period were examined. Research was facilitated by access to the *Republic*'s mainframe computer along with complete access to the archives at the *New Times.* The years 1986-1990 were chosen for this research because the archival database at the *Republic* only went back to 1986. Our data base is expanding yearly, and subsequent studies are forthcoming.

6. It has not been established absolutely that HIV/AIDS is *one* distinct biological—let alone social—phenomenon. This and other research confirms the existence of multiple social constructions of HIV/AIDS which have different parameters and consequences. These competing social constructions have been largely

presented by the media (Rappaport, 1988; Altman, 1986, pp. 38-39; Baker, 1986; Watney, 1989; & Plumer, 1989, pp. 20-51).

7. Kinsella attributes the *New York Times*'s initial lack of HIV/AIDS coverage to the homophobia of its then executive director, Abe Rosenthal (1990, pp. 59-60). He notes that later, however, Rosenthal became a kind of AIDS crusader, writing compassionate editorials on the issues of HIV/AIDS. The damage, unfortunately, had already been done.

8. "Presentable" has to do with time/space/length considerations as well as more substantive "content" issues, as determined by the editorial philosophy of a given news organization (Chancellor & Mears, 1983, p. 1-22).

9. For example, the American Heart Association, The American Cancer Association, the American Lung Association, among others, offer annual cash awards to reporters for "contributing to understanding of their field." These organizations continually supply health reporters with "press kits," organizational information, and programmatic agendas. The implication is that only reporters who portray the organization in a positive light will receive the organization-funded award.

10. The reason no HIV/AIDS stories appeared in the Phoenix *New Times* during 1989 is that the HIV/AIDS reporter was on sabbatical leave, while she wrote a book. Smaller papers, unfortunately, also have smaller budgets for reporters.

11. "Dominant type" refers to the single largest category of article, per year, in all HIV/AIDS-specific coverage examined.

12. "Medical/Scientific Updates" represent any stories concerning medical/ scientific developments related to the study and/or treatment of HIV/AIDS using specifically medical/biological discourse: e.g., discussions about the viral stamina of the HIV-virus and its meaning for the epidemic, discussions about the impact/ workings of AZT on the human immune system, and discussions of the progress of specific efforts of the "war" against HIV/AIDS.

13. "Public reaction" articles represent stories relating public perception or reaction to HIV/AIDS; e.g., polls on fear of AIDS, responses of local governmental officials to an HIV/AIDS "crisis"–how they plan to deal with an HIV-positive student in their school system, for example–or even how the federal government is dealing with the problems of HIV/AIDS. Much of this discourse also relied on medical/scientific testimony: e.g., a doctor's testimony about the likelihood of an HIV-positive student transmitting the virus to others. Articles like this comprised the single-largest category of article in 1987 and 1988 in the *Republic*.

REFERENCES

Albert, Edward. (1986). Illness and Deviance: The Response of the Press to AIDS. In D. Feldman & T. Johnson (Eds.), *The Social Dimensions of AIDS: Method and Theory*. New York: Praeger.
Altheide, David. (1976). *Creating Reality: How TV News Distorts Events*. Beverly Hills, CA: Sage.
Altheide, David. (1985). *Media Power*. Beverly Hills, CA: Sage.
Altheide, David, & Robert P. Snow. (1979). *Media Logic*. Beverly Hills, CA: Sage.

Altheide, David, & Robert P. Snow. (1991). *Media Worlds in the Postjournalism Era.* New York, NY: Aldine de Gruyter.

Altman, Dennis. (1986). *AIDS in the Mind of America.* Garden City, NY: Anchor Press/Doubleday.

Baker, Andrea J. (1986). The Portrayal of AIDS in the Media: An Analysis of Articles in the *New York Times.* In D. Feldman & T. Johnson (Eds.), *The Social Dimensions of AIDS: Method and Theory.* New York: Praeger.

Best, Joel (Ed.). (1989). *Images of Issues: Typifying Contemporary Social Problems.* New York: Aldine de Gruyter.

Chancellor, John, & Walter R. Mears. (1983). *The News Business.* New York: Mentor.

Conrad, Peter, & Joseph Schneider. (1980). *Deviance and Medicalization: From Badness to Sickness.* Toronto: The C.V. Mosby Company.

Ericson, Richard V., P. M. Baranek, & Janet B. L. Chan. (1989). *Negotiating Control: A Study of News Sources.* Toronto, Canada: University of Toronto Press.

Gilman, Sander. (1987). AIDS and Syphilis: The Iconography of Disease." *October, 43,* 87-108.

Gross, Larry. (1991). Out of the Mainstream: Sexual Minorities and the Mass Media. *Journal of Homosexuality, 21*(1/2), 19-46.

Keniston, Kenneth. (1990). Introduction to the Issue. In *Living with AIDS,* Stephen R. Graubard (Ed.). Cambridge: The MIT Press. pp. XVII-XL.

Kinsella, James. (1989). *Covering the Plague: AIDS and the American Media.* New Brunswick: Rutgers University Press.

Kitzinger, Jenny. (1990). Audience understandings of AIDS media messages: A discussion of methods. *Sociology of Health and Illness, 12*(3), 319-335.

Krippendorf, Klaus. (1980). *Content Analysis: An Introduction to Its Methodology.* Beverly Hills: Sage.

Plumer, Ken. (1988). Organizing AIDS. In *Social Aspects of AIDS,* Peter Aggleton and Hilary Homans (Eds.). New York: The Falmer Press.

Rappaport, Jon. (1988). *AIDS INC: Scandal of the Century.* San Bruno, CA: Human Energy Press.

Stipp, Horst, & Dennis Kerr. (1989). Determinants of Public Opinion About AIDS. *Public Opinion Quarterly, 53,* 98-106.

Thomas, Lewis. (1989). AIDS: A Long View. In *Public and Professional Attitudes Toward AIDS Patients: A National Dilemma,* David E. Rogers and Eli Ginzberg (Eds.). San Francisco: Westview Press.

Watney, Simon. (1989). The Subject of AIDS. In *AIDS: Social Representations, Social Practices,* Peter Aggleton, Graham Hart, & Peter Davies (Eds.). New York: The Falmer Press. 64-73.

Watney, Simon. (1988). AIDS, 'Moral Panic' Theory and Homophobia. In *Social Aspects of AIDS,* Peter Aggleton & Hilary Homans (Eds.). New York: The Falmer Press, 52-64.

Watney, Simon. (1987a). *Policing Desire. Pornography, AIDS and the Media.* London: Comedia, Methuen & Co. Ltd.

Watney, Simon. (1987). The Spectacle of AIDS. *October, 43,* 71-86.

Truth and Deception in AIDS Information Brochures

Austin Jones, PhD

Arizona State University

SUMMARY. This essay documents state governmental subversion of expansive constructions of HIV-disease. While it is clear that governments frequently practice deception and secrecy with the justification that the public would become dangerously emotional and irrational if fully informed, there is no evidence that the public would, in fact, behave that way. The essay concludes with a ranking of state AIDS brochures for accuracy and totality of information.

HIV disease and its terminal stage AIDS have been more extensively–and destructively–politicized in the United States than any other disease in the nation's history. This unfortunate phenomenon appears to have two principal sources. The first is the early and continuing stigmatization of AIDS as a disease of homosexual and

Austin Jones is Professor of Psychology at Arizona State University and President of the National Council on HIV-Disease. The National Council on HIV-Disease may be contacted at P.O. Box 66966, Phoenix, AZ 85082.

This article first appeared in *National Parents' Council on AIDS Quarterly Bulletin*, Fall 1993, and is reprinted here with permission. (The current name of the NPCA is National Council on HIV-Disease.)

[Haworth co-indexing entry note]: "Truth and Deception in AIDS Information Brochures." Jones, Austin. Co-published simultaneously in *Journal of Homosexuality* (The Haworth Press, Inc.) Vol. 32, No. 3/4, 1997, pp. 37-75; and: *Activism and Marginalization in the AIDS Crisis* (ed: Michael A. Hallett) The Haworth Press, Inc., 1997, pp. 37-75; and: *Activism and Marginalization in the AIDS Crisis* (ed: Michael A. Hallett) Harrington Park Press, an imprint of The Haworth Press, Inc., 1997, pp. 37-75.

bisexual men, although it was known by 1984 that AIDS in Africa and many other regions affected mostly heterosexual men and women. Encouraged by—and sometimes encouraging—the antagonism felt by much of the public toward homosexuals, many conservative leaders found in the HIV epidemic both a basis for renewed attacks upon the gay community, and justification for opposing federal funding for AIDS programs.

The second source of the politicization of HIV disease arose more gradually, is ever increasing, and is at this moment enormously more potent than previously—the perception on the part of top political leaders that the HIV epidemic is a public health catastrophe of such gargantuan scale that no amount of federal money and political skill can fix it, at least not within the relatively short periods of time to which politicians feel they must limit their attention in order to survive. This perception may indeed be well-rooted in reality, in view of the estimated cumulative total of five million HIV disease cases in the U.S. by the end of the decade; thus it is understandable that most political leaders are immobilized by apprehension and a sense of futility. As the National Commission on AIDS observed in its 1991 report *America Living with AIDS*, "The lack of government leadership is everywhere evident."

While the annual rates of AIDS continue to rise, especially among heterosexual women and teenagers, in 1992 the overall federal funding for AIDS-related programs was virtually unchanged, in constant dollars, from the previous year. After more than a decade, there is still no national plan for responding to the epidemic. At the highest levels of government, the characteristic response to the HIV epidemic continues to be denial of its seriousness and avoidance of thinking about it.

When wars go badly—and this lop-sided war between humanity and HIV is going very badly indeed—governments have traditionally been loath to broadcast the bleak news to the citizens, lest confidence in the governments themselves falter. A skirmish won is portrayed as a turning point in the war, plans for action are reported as certain to be successful, and when all appears hopeless, the public may never be told, but left unprepared to experience the consequences of defeat first-hand.

AIDS information brochures distributed to the public serve,

potentially, at least three critical functions in the war with HIV; these are the efforts to (1) prevent HIV infection, (2) control the public's emotional reaction to information about progress–or the lack of it–in the war with HIV, and (3) influence the public's cultural interpretation of the epidemic.

The first function is the publicly-stated or *declaratory* function of virtually all AIDS information brochures. The prevention of HIV infection is almost always approached from the standpoint of primary cause, principally sexual contact, shared needle usage, and the receipt of contaminated blood or blood products. (There are rare references to such indirect or secondary causal factors as poor nutrition and other factors which may weaken the immune system and increase the risk of infection.)

Functions (2) and (3) are never, it appears, declaratory, but even a quick reading of a small sample of AIDS information brochures suggests that they are important *operational* functions, though not explicitly identified. Regarding the second function, it is at least understandable–and perhaps rational in the short term–for governmental agencies to seek to control the level of fearful arousal elicited by public messages about the war with HIV, and to foster confidence in the agency issuing the information. Similarly, it should not be surprising that efforts to influence the cultural interpretation of the epidemic are apparent in many AIDS brochures–especially the perception of who, or what, is to blame.

With these thoughts in mind, the NPCA undertook a study of the AIDS information brochures distributed by state departments of health, in order to assess the adequacy of information provided concerning critical and politically sensitive aspects of the generally-held medical model of AIDS. While there are clearly some political sensitivities to the manner in which the prevention of infection is communicated, usually the declaratory function of the brochures, the study reported here focused upon the brochures' treatment of information related to the operational but rarely identified functions of controlling the public's fearful response and influencing its cultural interpretation of the epidemic.

THE GENERALLY HELD MEDICAL MODEL OF AIDS

In the United States, with a very few exceptions, virtually all medical researchers hold to a model of AIDS which includes the following four propositions:

1. *The continuity of HIV infection and AIDS.* AIDS is the terminal stage of a single, slowly-unfolding disease process which begins with HIV infection, and which is characterized by the progressive weakening of the immune system by HIV. (That AIDS is a consequence of HIV infection is now no longer treated by the Centers for Disease Control (CDC) as an empirical proposition but rather as a matter of definition: the diagnosis of AIDS requires either direct or presumptive evidence of HIV infection.)

2. *The near certainty that HIV infection will result in AIDS.* While the incubation period is highly variable, the probability is extremely high (i.e., it approaches 1.0 very closely) that HIV infection will eventually cause AIDS, unless medical treatments not yet discovered or death from other causes should intervene.

3. *The lethality of AIDS.* Although the life expectancy of individuals diagnosed with AIDS is highly variable, the probability is extremely high (i.e., it approaches 1.0 very closely) that AIDS will eventually cause death, unless medical treatments not yet discovered or death from other causes should intervene.

4. *The importance of behavior rather than group membership in determining the risk of HIV infection.* The sexual transmission of HIV is not determined by sexual orientation, but by sexual behavior. Unprotected sexual activity increases the risk of HIV infection for heterosexuals and homosexuals alike. There is no evidence that sexual orientation of itself is associated with either greater vulnerability to infection or greater risk of infecting others. Thus, the stigmatization of AIDS as a disease of homosexuals or other so-called high-risk groups is erroneous. Similarly, it is incorrect to stigmatize AIDS as a disease of Hispanics, African-Americans, or drug users, although each of these sub-populations currently experiences a disproportionately high rate of HIV infection.

HOW THE BROCHURES WERE SELECTED
AND EVALUATED

Letters were written in October 1991 to the departments of health of every state and the District of Columbia, requesting copies of the general information brochures on AIDS distributed to the public. For the purposes of this study, the term "general information brochure" refers to brochures which target the general public and which deal broadly with AIDS and HIV, rather than targeting such specific groups as IV drug users, teenagers, women, etc. General information brochures typically have titles like *What Everyone Should Know about AIDS* or *AIDS: Do You Know the Facts?*

Forty-seven states and the District of Columbia responded with a total of 72 different brochures which met the criteria for general information brochures. The brochures received from Arkansas and Wyoming did not meet the criteria, and none were received from Rhode Island. The majority were published by the state departments of health. In addition to state publications, many departments of health distributed brochures from the Centers for Disease Control, Surgeon General, American College Health Association, Red Cross, American Social Health Association, San Francisco AIDS Foundation, and Channing L. Bete. The domain of this study was limited to brochures of these publishers and those of the states.

Each brochure was evaluated for the adequacy of information provided concerning the four propositions of the generally-held medical model discussed above. The adequacy of information was judged with respect both to *accuracy* and *level of disclosure.* A preliminary review of the brochures revealed a startling degree of variability, ranging from accurate and relatively complete statements, to a complete absence of information and even to statements judged significantly misleading.

Each brochure was first rated for the amount of accurate information disclosed concerning the continuity of HIV infection and AIDS, the near certainty that HIV infection will result in AIDS, and the lethality of AIDS. A ten-point rating scale was employed, with scores ranging from −4 to +5. A rating of zero was given to brochures with no reference to the characteristic, with increasing positive values designating increasing amounts of information. A rating of +3 or above, defined as "excellent," was given to brochures which included a clear and substantially complete statement of the characteristic. A score greater than zero and less than 3 was given to brochures containing partial information and considered "adequate." Negative ratings were given to brochures which made statements judged factually erroneous or otherwise misleading, ranging from –1 (slightly misleading) to –4 (very seriously misleading).

Brochures were also rated for their emphasis on behavior rather than group membership in determining the risk of HIV infection. This characteristic was rated on a 5-point scale. Brochures countering stigmatization by placing emphasis on behavior rather than group membership were given a positive rating of 1 or 2. A neutral rating of zero identified brochures which neither fostered nor countered stigmatization, and ratings of –1 or –2 were given those which emphasized high-risk groups rather than high-risk behavior.

The criteria established for the highest-possible ratings for each of the four characteristics were as follows:

1. *Continuity of HIV infection and AIDS.* The brochure includes some form of statement that AIDS results from HIV infection, a description of the process by which infection results in a weakening of the immune system, and an explanation of the temporal characteristics of HIV infection (e.g., that it is usually a matter of years before acute illness occurs).
2. *The near certainty that HIV infection will result in AIDS.* The brochure includes a statement to the effect that HIV infection is believed to result eventually in AIDS in all, or nearly all, cases unless effective medical treatments should be developed or death occurs from other causes; a statement of the average incubation period and its variability; and information on the positive effect of treatment and healthful lifestyle once one is infected with HIV.
3. *The lethality of AIDS.* The brochure includes a statement that AIDS is always or virtually always fatal, unless effective medical treatments should be developed or death occurs from other causes; an explanation of the variability in life expectancy following the diagnosis of AIDS; and information on the positive effects of treatment and healthful lifestyle in prolonging life and enhancing its quality.

4. *The importance of behavior rather than group membership in determining the risk of HIV infection.* The brochure includes an explicit statement to the effect that the probability of infection is related to high-risk behavior rather than to group membership, and gives several examples.

Two judges read the 72 brochures independently and rated each on the four characteristics in accordance with the above criteria. There was a high degree of agreement between the judges, and their ratings were averaged to obtain the ratings reported below.

THE ADEQUACY OF INFORMATION PROVIDED IN THE BROCHURES

The Continuity of HIV Infection and AIDS

Of the four characteristics rated, the 72 brochures as a group were judged most effective in their information concerning the continuity of HIV infection and AIDS. Individual brochures received ratings ranging from 0 to +5, with a median of 2.0. Almost a third (31%) of the brochures were judged *excellent*, with ratings of +3 or greater, and about half (49%) were considered *adequate* (ratings greater than zero but less than 3). However, 21% of the brochures received a zero rating because they did not even mention HIV, or contained no clear statement that AIDS results from HIV. No brochures were assessed as misleading for this characteristic.

Figure 1 shows the adequacy of information provided concerning the continuity of HIV infection and AIDS. Clearly this characteristic is being covered fairly well in the brochures distributed by state departments of health, as 80% contain sufficient information to merit a positive rating.

The highest-rated presentations of the continuity of HIV infection and AIDS were contained in the brochures published by the American College Health Association (distributed by Maryland and West Virginia) and the American Council on Science and Health (distributed by Vermont), and in the state-published brochures of Alabama, Delaware, and Oregon.

The Delaware brochure titled *AIDS. Know the Facts. Be Safe.* (which received one of the highest combined ratings for all four characteristics) expresses the continuity of HIV infection and AIDS simply and succinctly:

> *AIDS–Acquired Immune Deficiency Syndrome.* It is a disease caused by a virus called HIV (Human Immunodeficiency Virus) that can destroy the body's ability to fight off illness. AIDS allows other infections into the body. These infections can kill. . . . The time between infection with HIV and a diagnosis of AIDS averages 8-10 years for adults, although the time is shorter for children.

Fifteen of the total sample of 72 brochures received zero ratings for the continuity of HIV infection and AIDS. Eleven of these were published by the states and the District of Columbia, three by the CDC, and one by Channing L. Bete. Each of the states, however, distributed at least one brochure receiving a positive rating. Seven different brochures published by the CDC were included in the sample, of which four received positive ratings. The most frequently distributed CDC brochure (eleven states), *HIV Infection and AIDS: Are You at Risk?*, received a weak positive rating of 1.

FIGURE 1. The continuity of HIV infection and AIDS: Ratings of information contained in the brochures.

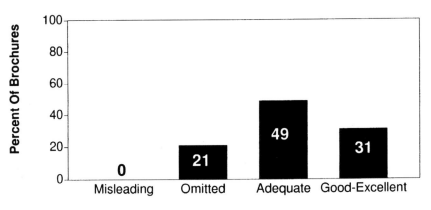

The highest-rated CDC brochure for this characteristic was *Voluntary HIV Counseling & Testing: Facts, Issues, and Answers*, which received a rating of 3.0. In addition to the brochure which received a zero rating, Channing L. Bete is the publisher of two brochures which received positive ratings.

The Near Certainty That HIV Infection Will Result in AIDS

The brochures received by far their lowest ratings for adequacy of information concerning the near certainty that HIV infection will result in AIDS. As shown in Figure 2, only 19% of the 72 brochures received positive ratings, while almost two-thirds (64%) were rated as misleading and received negative ratings—and an additional 18% provided no information at all.

The highest ratings (+4) were received by Michigan's *AIDS & Everyone* and the American College Health Association's *HIV Infection and AIDS*. Other highly-rated brochures were published by Delaware, the Red Cross, and the American Social Health Association.

In the Michigan brochure, as was true of all other brochures receiving a positive rating, the near certainty that HIV infection will

FIGURE 2. The near certainty that HIV infection will result in AIDS: Ratings of information contained in the brochures.

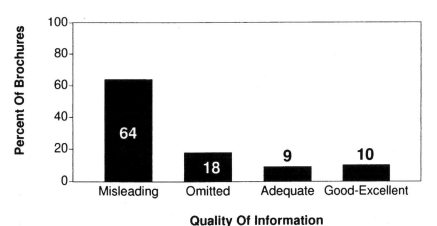

result in AIDS is expressed as a strong implication rather than as a direct statement:

> When a person becomes infected with HIV, it can be a number of years before any symptoms appear.

A similar approach is taken in the American College Health Association's brochure, which begins with the statement that "HIV causes a spectrum of conditions and symptoms." Beneath this statement is an illustration titled "The Spectrum of HIV Infection," consisting of a long horizontal rectangle colored pale blue at one end and gradually shading to dark blue at the other. Beneath the rectangle are the designations (from left to right) "infected . . . no symptoms . . . mild symptoms . . . AIDS." The text which follows includes these statements:

> People who have become infected with HIV may progress either slowly or quickly along the spectrum of HIV infection. . . . Given currently available information, it appears that, without treatment, most people will develop serious symptoms at some point in the future.

Within the group of brochures receiving negative ratings (46 out of the sample of 72) there were 14 rated –3.5 or –4.0 and judged *very seriously misleading*. There was considerable variability in the manner in which the statements rated as misleading were expressed. Representative of one sub-set is the simple factual-type statement in Montana's brochure *What Everyone Should Know about AIDS* (revised 1989):

> Presence of [HIV] antibodies means that a person has been infected with the virus but does *not* tell whether a person is still infected, has AIDS, or will ever develop AIDS.

This statement is clearly at odds with the present model of AIDS; a confirmed positive antibody test carries precisely the conclusion that the person *is* still infected and either has AIDS or is almost certain to get it in the future.

South Carolina's brochure *AIDS Information* (revised 1988) is similarly at variance with the current model of AIDS. Under the heading "What happens when a person gets the AIDS virus?" are the following statements:

Not everyone infected with the virus will develop AIDS.

- Many infected people will remain healthy, and show no symptoms of AIDS. The long-term effects of these people are not known. Some may be able to spread the virus to others.
- A smaller group of people will develop mild to severe illnesses that are called AIDS Related Complex (ARC).
- An even smaller group will develop AIDS.

The reason why these statements, like those of the Montana brochure, deviate so remarkably from the medical model of AIDS is not clear. While the expectation that all or nearly all HIV infections will result eventually in AIDS emerged gradually in the second half of the 1980s, by 1988 and 1989 (the respective dates of the South Carolina and Montana brochures), that view was sufficiently well established that a statement like "Many infected people will remain healthy and show no symptoms of AIDS" appears to have been more motivated to reassure, than to inform, the reader.

A somewhat different style of statement judged ambiguous and potentially misleading occurs in some brochures which include information about the average incubation period. The CDC's widely distributed 1991 brochure, *HIV Infection and AIDS: Are You at Risk?*, states:

About half of the people with HIV develop AIDS within 10 years, but the time between infection with HIV and the onset of AIDS can vary greatly.

For readers familiar with the expectation that HIV infection will almost certainly result eventually in AIDS it is clear that "the other half" of the people with HIV will take *longer* than 10 years to develop AIDS. But for the general public, the statement is likely to be taken to mean simply that "the other half" doesn't develop AIDS at all. The context in which the statement about the incubation period occurs can enhance the misleading implication. For example, the Arizona brochure *AIDS: Do You Know the Facts*, includes the following statement in a passage discussing HIV tests:

> If the test is positive, this means that the person has been infected with the virus. This does not mean that the person has AIDS or that they will develop AIDS. About 50% of infected individuals have developed AIDS within 10 years after being infected with HIV.

The sequence of the second and third sentences strongly implies that those who will *not* develop AIDS constitute the other 50% of those infected, and the passage was therefore judged seriously misleading.

The CDC brochures as a group received consistently low ratings for information about the near certainty that HIV infection will result in AIDS. Seven of the sample of 72 brochures were published by the CDC, and of those seven only one received a positive rating—the weakest positive rating given (+.5). Of the remaining six, two received zero ratings for absence of information and four received negative ratings ranging from –1 to –4 for statements judged misleading. The three Channing L. Bete brochures also received low ratings as a group (0., – 2. and –4). The influence of the CDC and Bete publications on the public perception of the epidemic is probably substantial; seventeen states and the District of Columbia distribute one or more of the seven CDC brochures reviewed in this study, and eight states distribute one or more of the three Bete brochures. (The total distribution of CDC and Bete brochures is, of course, much greater than these figures indicate, as they are also distributed by many organizations other than state departments of health.)

The adequacy of information about the near certainty that HIV infection will lead to AIDS is related to the publication date of the brochures, more recent brochures generally receiving higher ratings. Of the six highest-rated brochures, only one was published before 1990; three were published in 1990, and two in 1991. While several of the lowest-rated brochures were published in 1990 or 1991, publication years prior to 1989 are uniformly associated with the lowest rating (-4).

The significance of recency of publication is apparent in the brochures of the Red Cross and the Surgeon General. The three Red Cross brochures in the sample were published in 1986, 1988, and 1989. Their ratings were –4, 0 and +3, respectively, demonstrating a shift over that period from statements judged "very seriously misleading" to those judged "excellent." Similarly, the Surgeon General's 1986 brochure, *Surgeon General's Report on AIDS*, received a rating of –2 (moderately misleading), but the 1991 brochure *Understanding AIDS* received a +2 rating (adequate).

The Lethality of AIDS

With respect to the lethality of AIDS, approximately two-thirds of the brochures either omitted any discussion of lethality, or made statements judged misleading (Figure 3). Most misleading statements were rated in the slight-to-moderate range, with only 4% falling in the very seriously misleading range. Similarly, only 4% were judged excellent, with 29% falling in the adequate range.

Although there is near-universal agreement, within the public health and medical organizations which produced most of the brochures in this sample, that AIDS always or almost always leads to death, only four brochures included direct and unequivocal statements to that effect, receiving a rating of +4. Oregon's 1990 brochure *HIV/AIDS: Know the Facts* was judged especially effective in part because its statement of lethality is placed in the opening paragraph, headed "What Is AIDS?" The entire opening paragraph is quoted here:

FIGURE 3. The Lethality of AIDS: Ratings of information contained in the brochures.

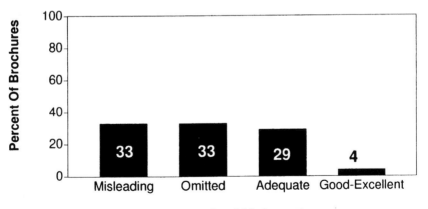

AIDS is short for Acquired Immunodeficiency Syndrome. AIDS is caused by infection from a virus known as HIV, Human Immunodeficiency Virus. The virus weakens the body's immune system to the point where the person can become infected by illnesses that usually don't affect healthy people. A form of cancer called Kaposi's Sarcoma, Pneumocystis carinii pneumonia, and infections caused by viruses, fungi, and parasites are a few of the illnesses AIDS patients can suffer. *AIDS leads to death.* (emphasis added)

The brochure reinforces the lethality of AIDS by the following statement which appears under the heading "How Is AIDS Treated":

There is no known cure for AIDS. Doctors treat AIDS patients for their specific infections or cancers. There are experimental drugs that will slow the progress of the disease. But no drug has yet been discovered that will kill HIV or repair the body's damaged immune system.

North Dakota published the brochure which is smallest in size, briefest in text, and most succinct in its statement of lethality: *AIDS IS FATAL.*

As this statement is not qualified in any way, it appears probable that most readers would interpret it to mean that AIDS is always fatal. Tennessee's *AIDS: What You Should Know* also contains a similarly blunt and unqualified statement as the first sentence of the brochure:

Acquired Immune Deficiency Syndrome (AIDS) is a currently fatal condition.

The only other publication in the sample which made a direct, unequivocal statement of lethality is the American Council on Science and Health's *Answers about AIDS.* This 1989 publication constitutes a special case in the sample because of its unusual length—it is a skillfully designed booklet of 53 pages. Its statement of lethality, like Oregon's, is prominently placed in the opening paragraph under the heading "AIDS: An Overview":

> AIDS, or acquired immunodeficiency syndrome, is a recently recognized condition caused by a virus that cripples the body's immune system, and leaves the person vulnerable to certain types of infections that do not occur, or produce only mild illness. in individuals with normal immune systems. *AIDS appears to be an invariably fatal illness* . . . (emphasis added)

While the length of the ACSH's booklet may limit its usefulness for distribution to the public, it was judged a contribution of exceptional quality, and will be discussed more fully later in this report.

The next most highly rated brochure (+3) was Delaware's "AIDS: Know the Facts. Be Safe.," in which the near-certainty that AIDS will result in death is expressed as a strong implication: "Once someone has AIDS, the average survival time is about two years; however, there are a small number of people with AIDS who live longer." In several brochures the statements regarding lethality were expressed as weaker implications, or contained ambiguous or inconsistent elements, and thus received somewhat lower positive ratings.

While 24 of the brochures were rated in some degree misleading regarding the lethality of AIDS, very few made statements judged to be factually incorrect. Rather, the impression that AIDS is less often lethal than is generally believed, was usually conveyed by an overall, mildly optimistic tone and/or by adverbs like "sometimes" and verbs such as "can kill" (rather than "will kill" or "does kill"). The raters found many of these brochures simply unclear in the passages which dealt with lethality, often rereading them many times in the effort to determine what, precisely, was being said. In many such instances, the question of lethality was unresolved, with the reader left to pick from the more pessimistic or more optimistic elements in a confusing passage. There is strong empirical evidence that in such ambiguous situations most readers will make the interpretation that is least fear-arousing.

Kentucky's brochure *What You Should Know about AIDS.* begins with a brief and seemingly direct statement which contains a significant ambiguity:

> What is AIDS?
> AIDS is the Acquired Immune Deficiency Syndrome–a serious illness which makes the body unable to fight infections. A

> person with AIDS is susceptible to certain infections and can-
> cers. When a person's body cannot fight off infections, they
> become ill and *sometimes* die. (emphasis added)

The ambiguity here lies in the word "sometimes," which could
be interpreted as referring to AIDS, with the meaning that one
sometimes dies of AIDS—not always or almost always. It was the
raters' opinion that this ambiguity leaves the reader with a more
optimistic feeling about surviving AIDS than if the passage had
been omitted altogether; the brochure was judged moderately misleading, with a rating of –2.

Similar ambiguity appears in Massachusetts' brochure *AIDS:
Learn and Live.* The opening sentences of the brochure state "Any
man or woman can get the AIDs virus. AIDS kills. We do not yet
have a cure." This statement, as it stands, is a relatively strong
expression of lethality, limited only by not having said, e.g.,
"invariably kills" or "kills in all or virtually all cases." Statements
in a subsequent paragraph, however, introduce significant elements
of ambiguity:

> AIDS is caused by a virus that can attack the body's defense
> system and block the ability to fight off other diseases and
> infections.
>
> If the defense system is only weakened, people may feel and
> look healthy. If the defense is severely damaged, people *may*
> become ill and die from AIDS. (emphasis added)

Despite the initial statement that "AIDS kills," the overall effect of
the several statements taken together is to mislead the reader by
implying that the lethality of AIDS is less than is almost universally
believed to be the case. The last sentence quoted above comes close
to, or is, a bald misstatement of fact. To say that persons with AIDS
whose defense systems are severely damaged *may* become ill and
die simply does not wash as a credible statement.

Pennsylvania's brochure, *Facts about AIDS*, provides a similar
example of the troublesome usage of the word "may":

> AIDS is a serious condition that destroys a person's natural
> immunity against infectious diseases and some forms of can-

cer. People with AIDS *may* get serious illnesses that are not a threat to someone whose immune system is working the right way. (emphasis added)

The usage of "may" in this passage suggests not only that many people with AIDS will not die, but also that many will not even get serious illnesses.

The otherwise exemplary brochure *HIV/AIDS* published by the American Social Health Association contains a statement judged misleading, in part because of the usage of the word "can":

People with AIDS experience certain life-threatening infections and cancers that make them very sick and *can* eventually kill them.
. . . Many people now consider HIV infection a manageable, long-term illness. (emphasis added)

In the first of these two sentences, the word "can" is, of course, in one sense factually accurate—people with AIDS do indeed experience infections and cancers that *can* (i.e., have the ability to) kill them. The problem lies in the fact that "can" carries the additional, connotative meaning of "might," making it easy for the reader to conclude that death is by no means the certain or near-certain outcome of AIDS. This interpretation is enhanced by the second sentence quoted above, which conveys a sense of optimism that is probably not warranted.

In the most widely distributed of the CDC's brochures, *HIV Infection and AIDS: Are You at Risk?*, a sense of optimism is conveyed both by portions of the text and by the numerous pictures of attractive people, many of them smiling and none frowning or looking sad. The 13-page brochure is beautifully designed and expensively printed—heavy coated paper, large type, handsome photographs, lots of white space. (The expression "puff-piece" comes to mind.) None of the 10 photographs (all of people) have a caption, and only three have a clear relationship to the text. The passages relevant to the question of lethality are as follows:

AIDS stands for acquired immunodeficiency syndrome, a disease in which the body's immune system breaks down. Normally, the immune system fights off infections and certain other diseases. When the system fails, a person with AIDS can develop a variety of life-threatening illnesses.

About half of the people with HIV develop AIDS within 10 years, but the time between infection with HIV and the onset of AIDS can vary greatly. The severity of the HIV-related illness or illnesses will differ from person to person, according to many factors, including the overall health of the individual.

Today there are promising new medical treatments that can postpone many of the illnesses associated with AIDS. This is a step in the right direction, and scientists are becoming optimistic that HIV infection will someday be controllable. In the meantime, people who get medical care to monitor and treat their HIV infection can carry on with their lives, including their jobs, for longer than ever before.

Each of these three paragraphs, examined literally, is technically correct in terms of the generally accepted model of AIDS, yet each appears to have been written with the goal of reassuring the reader that being infected with HIV or having AIDS isn't all *that* bad, and that, in any case, research in medical treatment is advancing rapidly. Nowhere in the entire brochure do the "D" or "F" words (death, deadly, die, fatal) ever occur, not even once. In the first paragraph, the use of "can" and "threatening" suggests that persons with AIDS *might* not develop such illnesses and that they are *not necessarily* deadly when they do occur.

It is doubtful that most of the public would read the second paragraph with the same understanding of those who wrote it. The first sentence can easily be interpreted as meaning that the *other half* of the people with HIV (i.e., who *don't* develop AIDS within 10 years) simply *never* develop it. This interpretation is not nearly so scary as the conclusion that HIV infection always or virtually always leads to AIDS. Further reassurance is given by the statement that the severity of the "HIV-related illness or illnesses" varies in accordance with many factors including the individual's overall health. The avoidance of the word AIDS in this sentence is part of its essential ambiguity–readers who are not seriously ill can easily imagine themselves not likely to die even if infected.

The third paragraph is perhaps even more selective in its reassuring phrases. If you have AIDS or should get it in the future, not to worry; the language of the brochure is soothing–". . . promising new medical treatments . . . step in the right direction . . . can carry on with their lives . . . longer than ever before." This paragraph is remarkable for its discussion of a lethal process in such a way as to render its lethality all but invisible. Because of the consistent pattern of ambiguity coupled with reassurance, the brochure as a whole was judged seriously misleading and received a rating of –3.

The Importance of Behavior Rather Than Group Membership in Determining the Risk of HIV Infection

The stigmatization of persons with AIDS is expressed principally in an emphasis on high-risk groups rather than high-risk behavior. The stigmatization of AIDS as a mostly homosexual disease continues to fade, but only slowly. Less than half the brochures (41%) received positive ratings for emphasizing behavior rather than group membership in determining the risk of HIV infection (Figure 4). Thirty percent received negative ratings because of their emphasis on membership in high-risk groups, and 28% were judged neutral with respect to stigmatization, neither reinforcing nor opposing it.

The three brochures most highly rated for an emphasis on behavior rather than group membership are those of Michigan, Tennessee, and the American College Health Association. In Michigan's brochure *AIDS & Everyone*, the issue of stigmatization is addressed in the third paragraph, prominently located on page one:

> Some people still believe that only people in certain "high risk groups" can become infected with HIV. This is not true. *Who you are* has nothing to do with whether you are at risk of HIV infection. What matters is *what you do*. (Italicized phrases appear in bold print in the brochure.)

On page two, the counter-stigmatizing message is contained in the first sentence under the heading "How Do You Get Infected from Sex?":

HIV can be spread by sexual intercourse whether you are a male or female, heterosexual, homosexual, or bisexual.

Tennessee's *AIDS and Sex: What You Should Know,* also addresses the issue of stigmatization in statements that are blunt and well-positioned:

Who Gets AIDS?

Anyone can get AIDS. In Tennessee, both gay and straight people have AIDS. Men and women have it. About half the babies born to infected mothers have the virus. These children usually die within three years. People of all races can get AIDS if they don't know how to protect themselves.

In short, *anyone* can get AIDS.

What Kind of Sex Spreads HIV?

Intercourse (penetration) is the main way HIV is spread. Intercourse can be vaginal or anal and can be between two men, a man and woman or between two women.

FIGURE 4. The importance of behavior rather than group membership in determining the risk of HIV infection: Ratings of information contained in the brochures in terms of emphasis on behavior or group membership.

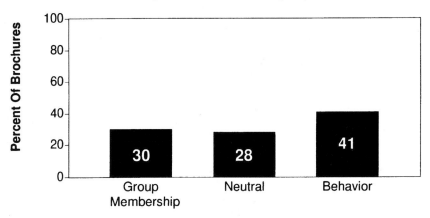

Both the Michigan and (especially) the Tennessee brochures employ a vocabulary and literary style well suited for wide distribution to people of varied educational level. The American College Health Association's *HIV Infection and AIDS* is a well-designed, longer brochure written at a level more suited for people with college education. This brochure addresses the issue of stigmatization in several passages, the first of which is titled "It's What You Do, Not Who You Are":

> It's what you do, not who you are, that matters in HIV infection. "Risk behaviors" are much more important than "risk groups." Anyone who engages in unsafe sexual behavior or shares needles for any reason can become infected with HIV. HIV can be transmitted during sexual intercourse among people who define themselves as gay, bisexual, or straight. HIV can be transmitted during needle sharing by people who may or may not be "addicted" to drugs. . . .

> Some people know a great deal about HIV and AIDS. But people "in the know" still acquire HIV infection. A lot of people think HIV infection is a problem for "other" kinds of people in "other" places, and they feel invulnerable. But behaviors, not groups, transmit HIV.

The brochure also includes effective counter-stigmatizing information concerning HIV infection in racial minorities and women, and a particularly important statement designed to counter the self-stigmatization of many gay and bisexual men. No other brochure in the sample addresses the issues of stigmatization in as systematic and enlightening way.

Most of the 22 brochures with negative ratings included a section titled "Who Gets AIDS?" "Who Is Likely to Get AIDS?," or some similar wording, followed by a listing of risk groups beginning with homosexual and bisexual men. Florida's brochure *AIDS Information* is perhaps the most patently stigmatizing, in part because of the choice of the heading:

Risk Groups

There are some groups of people who stand a greater chance of contracting AIDS than others. These include:

- Gay or bisexual men
- I.V. drug users
- Hemophiliacs
- Sex partners of people in these groups
- Sex partners of someone with HIV infection, ARC, or AIDS

North Dakota's *AIDS Facts* and South Carolina's *Facts about . . . AIDS* contain similar listings of risk groups. The remaining 19 brochures received lesser negative ratings because their stigmatizing elements were weaker or placed less prominently.

The use of out-of-date brochures appears to be related particularly to the inclusion of stigmatizing passages. For example, the above-noted brochures of Florida, North Dakota, and South Carolina were published in 1987, 1988, and 1988 respectively. Failure to revise them prior to distribution in 1991 is a deficiency seen in many other brochures as well.

OVERALL RATINGS OF BROCHURES

For each brochure, the ratings for the four characteristics evaluated in this study were averaged to determine a composite score. Table 1 shows the ranking of the brochures, identified by publisher, with the educational level for which the brochures appear most appropriate. Tied ranks were assigned to those brochures receiving identical composite scores. Table 1 also includes a recommendation for each brochure as *highly recommended, acceptable,* or *not recommended,* often qualified by *with revision,* or *with other literature* (i.e., only if accompanied by additional literature in order to provide more comprehensive information). The qualification *with revision* refers to the need for only minor revision. Brochures considered acceptable only with extensive revision are designated simply as *not recommended.*

The percents of brochures receiving the various categories of recommendation are shown in Figure 5. While 82% of the brochures received some form of positive recommendation, only 5.6% (four brochures) were highly recommended as is. Eighteen percent were not recommended.

While the composite scores and the ranking of the brochures were derived exclusively from the ratings of the four characteristics studied, the recommendations take other considerations into account also. This was done in order to provide recommendations which would be of greatest practical usefulness. As a consequence, some brochures with the same ranking received different recommendations because of differences in the quality of information on topics other than the four characteristics which were the focus of this study.

The top-ranked brochures are very good indeed, and provide models which should be emulated widely. The highest-ranked brochure, the American Council on Science and Health's *Answers about AIDS*, is a special case because of its length—53 pages—and the high educational level required of its readers. The text is consistently outstanding, but appears readily accessible only to readers educated in the upper half of U.S. colleges and universities. Despite this limitation, it has great value for those with strong educational backgrounds and is also an excellent resource for HIV educators.

Ranked second (first among the state-published brochures) is Delaware's *AIDS: Know the facts and be safe*, followed closely by the Red Cross' *HIV Infection and AIDS*, the American College Health Association's *HIV Infection and AIDS*, Michigan's *AIDS and Everyone*,"and Tennessee's *AIDS and Sex: What You Should Know*—all of which are highly recommended, either as is or with minor revisions.

While the landmark (1986) *Surgeon General's Report on AIDS* is out of date in several respects and therefore not recommended now, the 1991 brochure, *Understanding AIDS*, which was prepared by the Surgeon General and the CDC, is among the top-ranked (11th) and highly recommended with minor revision.

Three of the four lowest-ranked brochures, each judged *not recommended*, are Georgia's *The Facts: AIDS*, South Carolina's *The Facts About . . .* (sic), and the CDC's *HIV Infection and AIDS: Are You at Risk?* The fourth, *recommended with revision*, is the San Francisco AIDS Foundation's *Straight Talk about Sex and AIDS*. The seven CDC brochures included in this study ranged from the highly-ranked (16th) *Understanding AIDS Fact Sheet* (highly recommended with minor revision) to the bottom-ranked *HIV infection and AIDS: Are You at Risk?* (not recommended). Five of the seven CDC brochures fall in the lower half of the rankings.

TABLE 1. Ranking of Brochures

Rank	Publisher	Title	Composite Score	Date Published	Education Level	Recommendation
1	Am Council on Science & Health	Answers about AIDS	3.5	7/89	Coll+	high rec as is
2	Delaware	AIDS: Know the Facts and be Safe	3.1	11/90	HS+ & Coll	high rec as is
3	Red Cross	HIV Infection and AIDS	3.0	5/89	All	high rec as is
4.5	Am College Health Association	HIV Infection and AIDS	2.5	1990	Coll+	high rec w/ rev
4.5	Michigan	AIDS and Everyone	2.5	no date	HS+ & Coll	high rec w/ rev
6	Tennessee	AIDS and Sex: What you should know	2.4	7/89	HS+ & Coll	high rec as is
7.5	Tennessee	AIDS: What you should know	1.4	7/89	HS+ & Coll	high rec w/ rev
7.5	Iowa	Facts about AIDS	1.4	no date	All	rec w/ other lit
11	Am Social Health Association	HIV/AIDS–Questions/Answers	1.2	1991	Coll+	high rec w/ rev
11	New Jersey	AIDS Risk: A Reference Guide	1.2	1987	HS+ & Coll	rec w/ other lit
11	Alabama	AIDS/HIV: What you should know	1.2	8/90	HS & Coll	rec w/ rev
11	Texas	What Everyone Should Know About AIDS & HIV	1.2	1/91	All	high rec w/ rev
11	Surgeon General	Understanding AIDS	1.2	1991	HS+ & Coll	high rec w/ rev
14.5	New York	AIDS: 100 Questions and Answers	1.0	7/91	HS+ & Coll	high rec w/ rev
14.5	Red Cross	Children, Parents, and AIDS	1.0	11/88	All	high rec w/ rev

		Title	Score	Date	Level	Recommendation
16	CDC	Understanding AIDS (fact sheet)	0.9	7/91	HS+ & Coll	high rec w/ rev
18	Hawaii	AIDS Information	0.8	7/91	HS+ & Coll	not recommended
18	Oregon	AIDS: Gathering the Facts	0.8	no date	Coll+	rec w/ rev
18	Missouri	25 Questions People Ask About AIDS	0.8	4/91	HS+ & Coll	rec w/ rev
21.5	Illinois	AIDS Facts for Life—Antibody Testing	0.6	2/91	HS+ & Coll	rec w/ rev
21.5	Alabama	Facts about AIDS	0.6	8/90	Coll	acceptable w/ rev
21.5	Alabama	Don't Die With AIDS—Live With Facts	0.6	4/90	All	acceptable w/ rev
21.5	Colorado	AIDS: The Sexually Active Heterosexual	0.6	3/91	All	rec w/ rev
25.5	Am College Health Association	AIDS—What Everyone Should Know	0.5	1987	Coll	rec w/ rev
25.5	Massachusetts	You and Your Family: Protect Yourself Against AIDS. It's Easy	0.5	no date	All	rec w/ other lit
25.5	Virginia	AIDS Information That Everyone Ought to Know	0.5	no date	HS+ & Coll	rec w/ other lit w/ rev
25.5	Channing L. Bete	What Everyone Should Know About AIDS	0.5	1991	HS	rec w/ rev
29	San Francisco AIDS Foundation	Fact vs. Fiction: Ten Things You Should Know About AIDS	0.4	no date	HS+ & Coll	rec w/ other lit w/ rev
29	Minnesota	AIDS Facts	0.4	1/91	Coll	high rec w/ rev
29	Illinois	Facts for Life—Answers to the 10 Most Frequently Asked Questions About AIDS	0.4	7/90	HS+ & Coll	rec w/ rev
32.5	Channing L. Bete	About AIDS	0.2	1991	HS	rec w/ rev
32.5	Colorado	Questions and Answers About AIDS	0.2	3/91	HS+ & Coll	rec w/ rev
32.5	Ohio	You Don't Have to Get AIDS	0.2	2/90	All	rec w/ rev

Rank	Publisher	Title	Composite Score	Date Published	Education Level	Recommendation
32.5	CDC	Voluntary HIV Counseling & Testing: Facts, Issues, and Answers	0.2	no date	HS+ & coll	rec. w/ rev
35.5	Maine	AIDS: Am I at Risk?	0.1	8/91	All	high rec w/ rev
35.5	Pennsylvania	Questions and Answers about AIDS	0.1	12/90	All	rec w/ rev
41	New York	AIDS: Facts About Acquired Immune Deficiency Syndrome	0.0	9/88	HS+ & Coll	rec w/ rev
41	Am Social Health Association	AIDS: Questions, Answers	0.0	3/88	HS+ & Coll	rec w/ rev
41	Missouri	Will I get AIDS— Answers to Important Questions	0.0	1989	All	acceptable w/ other lit
41	Montana	What Everyone Should Know About AIDS	0.0	4/89	HS+ & Coll	high rec w/ rev
41	North Dakota	AIDS – What you can do	0.0	10/88	HS & Coll	not recommended
41	Wisconsin	AIDS – What is it?	0.0	12/89	All	acceptable w/ other lit w/ rev
41	Wisconsin	AIDS: Why Take Chances?	0.0	12/89	All	high rec w/ rev
41	CDC	How You Won't Get AIDS	0.0	4/91	All	rec w/ other lit
41	CDC	AIDS & You	0.0	1989	All	acceptable w/ other lit

47	San Francisco AIDS Foundation	AIDS Lifeline: The Best Defense Against AIDS is Information	–0.1	1989	All	rec w/ rev
47	Idaho	Facts About AIDS in Idaho	–0.1	12/90	HS+ & Coll	rec w/ rev
47	Kentucky	What You Should Know about AIDS	–0.1	3/91	All	rec w/ rev
51	New York	AIDS: What Everyone Should Know	–0.2	8/87	All	not recommended
51	Indiana	HIV/AIDS Information for the General Public	–0.2	no date	All	rec w/ rev
51	Oregon	HIV/AIDS: Know the Facts	–0.2	4/90	HS+ & Coll	rec w/ rev
51	Surgeon General	Surgeon General's Report on AIDS	–0.2	10/22/86	Coll	not recommended
51	Washington D.C.	AIDS: The More We Know, the Less We Have to Fear	–0.2	no date	HS+ & Coll	acceptable w/ rev
56	Channing L. Bete	About Protecting Yourself from AIDS	–0.5	1991	HS	rec w/ rev
56	South Carolina	AIDS Information The best defense against AIDS	–0.5	7/88	HS+ & Coll	not recommended
56	West Virginia	Facts About AIDS	–0.5	no date	HS+ & Coll	acceptable w/ rev
56	CDC	What About AIDS Testing?	–0.5	1988	HS+ & Coll	rec w/ rev
56	CDC	What You Should Know About AIDS	–0.5	no date	All	acceptable w/ rev
59.5	Massachusetts	AIDS: Learn and Live	–0.6	no date	All	rec w/ rev
59.5	Arizona	AIDS – Do You Know The Facts?	–0.6	5/91	HS+ & Coll	rec w/ rev
61	Massachusetts	Should You Be Tested?	–0.8	no date	All	rec w/ rev
62	Illinois	Their Past Could Make You History	–0.9	3/90	HS+ & Coll	not recommended

Rank	Publisher	Title	Composite Score	Date Published	Education Level	Recommendation
63	New Hampshire	What is the Test? AIDS	−1.0	no date	HS+ & Coll	rec w/ rev
64	Red Cross	Latest Facts About AIDS: If Your Test for Antibody to the AIDS Virus is Positive	−1.1	10/86	HS+ & Coll	not recommended
65.5	North Dakota	AIDS Facts	−1.4	8/88	All	not recommended
65.5	North Carolina	What Everyone Should Know About AIDS	−1.4	10/89	HS+ & Coll	not recommended
67	Florida	AIDS Information	−1.5	9/87	HS+ & Coll	not recommended
68	Pennsylvania	Facts About AIDS	−1.6	12/90	HS+ & Coll	not recommended
70.5	CDC	HIV Infection and AIDS: Are You at Risk?	−1.8	5/91	All	not recommended
70.5	Georgia	The Facts: AIDS	−1.8	8/89	HS+ & Coll	not recommended
70.5	San Francisco AIDS Foundation	Straight Talk About Sex and AIDS	−1.8	1987	All	rec w/ rev
70.5	South Carolina	The Facts About . . .	−1.8	7/88	All	not recommended

* Tied ranks were assigned to those brochures receiving identical composite scores. Under *Educational Level*, the designations of *HS* and *Coll* refer to the lower half of high school and colleges with respect to academic standards, and the designations of *HS+* and *Coll+* refer to the upper half. In the *Recommendation* column, brochures are designated as *highly recommended as is* (i.e., without revision), *highly recommended with revision*, *recommended with other literature*, (i.e., recommended only if accompanied by additional literature), *acceptable with revisions*, *acceptable with other literature* (i.e., accompanied by additional literature), and *not recommended.*

While the composite score and the ranking of the brochures were derived exclusively from the ratings of the four characteristics studied, the recommendations take other considerations into account also. This was done in order to provide recommendations which would be of greatest practical usefulness. As a consequence, some brochures with the same ranking received different recommendations because of differences in the quality of information on topics other than the four characteristics which were the focus of this study.

FIGURE 5. Overall recommendation of brochures.

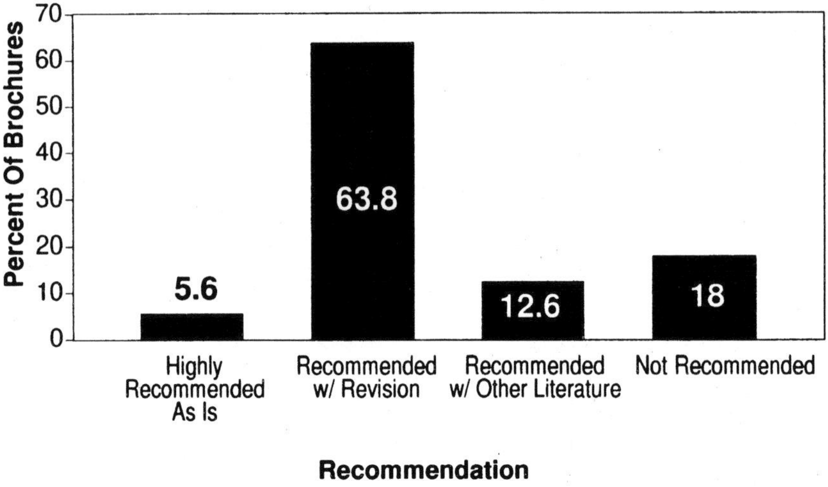

Recommendation

TRUTH AND DECEPTION

The widespread occurrence of misleading statements in AIDS information brochures raises several disturbing questions. Eighty-four percent of the brochures contained one or more statements judged misleading with respect to critical aspects of the generally-held medical model of AIDS–and in every instance, the effect of the misleading statement is to foster the perception that HIV infection and AIDS are less dangerous than almost all medical researchers believe them to be.

What accounts for such a high frequency of misinformation? Is it plausible that the misleading statements arose mostly through igno-rance or carelessness–or does deception appear to be involved? Or, perhaps, do statements judged misleading simply reflect honest differences of opinion within the scientific community?

The last of these questions can be easily answered "no." While there is a very small number of scientists who dispute the generally-held model of AIDS, there is no indication that any of them influenced the way the brochures were written. Rather, the bro-chures were prepared by the various state departments of health and the CDC, or by organizations such as the Red Cross and the American College Health Association, which share their viewpoints.

The hypothesis that most of the misleading statements reflect either ignorance or carelessness by the writers can be discounted almost as quickly. While it is not inconceivable that some writers were ill-informed or careless—and that their colleagues and superiors failed to detect this before printing—the sheer frequency of the misleading statements argues against such an interpretation. Also arguing against it is the substantial similarity of the misleading statements in many of the brochures. While it is theoretically possible that large numbers of writers might express ignorance or carelessness in very similar ways, the probability of such an outcome appears vanishingly small. The fact that all misleading statements, without exception, understated the danger of HIV infection and/or AIDS, makes it all the more difficult to attribute the similarity of the misleading statements to chance alone.

The evidence strongly suggests, but does not prove, that the widespread inclusion of misleading statements in AIDS information brochures represents the systematic practice of deception in order to control the public's emotional reaction to the epidemic. This is a serious matter. Yet surely no ordinarily observant citizen would be startled by the notion that governments frequently attempt to shape public attitude by substantial distortions of the truth. Indeed, lying to the public has become such a commonplace activity that the euphemism "disinformation" is widely employed to designate lying carried out by governments and governmental agencies; individual citizens may "lie," but governments only "disinform."

Deception is usually defined as making a person believe what is not true, and *lying* as making a statement one knows to be false with the intent to deceive. The invariability with which the misleading statements in the brochures understate the danger of HIV infection and AIDS as held by the generally-accepted medical model of AIDS, suggests that deceiving and lying to the public about AIDS have become routine.

Probable motives for deceiving the public about the HIV epidemic are easy to discern. The damage to both the nation's health care system and its overall economy will be catastrophic if the epidemic continues unchecked along its present course. The federal government appears, understandably if regrettably, to be immobilized by anxiety over its premonition that vast sums of money will be required to cope with the epidemic and that success is by no means assured. The characteristic response of the government to the epidemic continues to be denial of its seriousness and avoidance of thinking about it. What political leaders fear even more than the catastrophe of the epidemic itself is the anticipated reaction of the public when it realizes that the epidemic is not under control, and that no national plan exists for helping the health care system deal with its impact.

A further motive for deceiving the public about the epidemic can be inferred from the continued prominence of statements in the brochures which foster the misconception that HIV infection and AIDS are closely related to membership in "high-risk groups" rather than to risky behavior. The largely successful efforts to stigmatize AIDS as a disease of homosexuals, IV drug addicts, and other "marginalized" groups can be seen as an expression of governmental efforts to control the public's cultural interpretation of the epidemic. Should the epidemic proceed along its present calamitous path, better that the public's anger be directed to stigmatized groups rather than to the nation's political leadership.

Motivation to restrict the public's knowledge of the epidemic is evident also in lying's close cousin, secrecy. Former Surgeon General Koop states in his memoirs that throughout the first Reagan administration, he was forbidden by the White House even to mention AIDS in a public meeting. In the second Reagan administration, that ban was lifted but other efforts to control information about AIDS continued. At least through 1988, important scientific reports on HIV and AIDS were submitted by the CDC for review and editing to the Domestic Policy Council before being released to the public.

More subtle than secrecy, the public's access to critical information can be restricted by the decision not even to acquire the information in the first place. Thus, early in the epidemic, the decision was made by the CDC not to acquire systematic, nationwide sampling data on the prevalence of HIV infection. Thus, only "AIDS" could be counted, rather than the far greater number of those infected with HIV, although HIV infection is believed to result always or virtually always in AIDS. In this manner both the public and political leaders are denied access to critical data—not because of secrecy, but because it isn't there.

Can governmental efforts to deceive the public about the HIV epidemic be justified? Sissela Bok, in her highly-regarded book *Lying: Moral Choice in Public and Private Life*, notes that the most prominent excuses for lying invoke a moral principle. First among them are the principles of *avoiding harm* and *producing benefit*, and both appear to underlie the misleading statements in AIDS information brochures. Though rarely if ever expressed in print, the view is sometimes discussed privately that full public disclosure of information about the epidemic would diminish hope and cause panic. By giving some measure of false reassurance to the public, and withholding certain information, substantial harm is avoided. And by fostering calmness and optimism, great benefits are produced; the public is thereby made more cooperative and tolerant of the lack of progress in checking the epidemic.

Especially compelling as a justification for lying, in the view of governments and individuals alike, is the conviction that a crisis exists where only deception can prevent overwhelming harm. Bok develops this point in the following passage:

At times, those who govern also regard particular circumstances as too uncomfortable, too painful, for most people to be able to cope with rationally. They may believe, for instance, that their country must prepare for long-term challenges of great importance, such as a war, an epidemic, or a belt-tightening in the face of future shortages. Yet they may fear that citizens will be able to respond only to short-range dangers. Deception at such times may seem to the government leaders as the only means of attaining the necessary results.

Bok believes that lying in such circumstances can be justified only very rarely, if ever:

The fact that rare circumstances exist where the justification for government lying seems powerful creates a difficulty—these same excuses will often be made to serve a great many more purposes. For some governments or public officials, the information they wish to conceal is almost never of the requisite certainty, the time never the right one, and the public never sufficiently dispassionate.

What criteria exist by which government deception could be morally justified? Such criteria exist, Bok argues, but are very difficult to satisfy. The two principal criteria are those of *publicity* and the *assent of reasonable persons*. The criterion of publicity requires that the justification be given a public statement and a public defense. Thus, no secret moral justification could satisfy the criterion of publicity. The criterion of the assent of reasonable persons requires the agreement not only of the liar's friends and colleagues, but also of all those reasonable persons who will be affected by the lie, including those lied to. These criteria need not be applied to a specific deception, but must be satisfied *in advance* with respect to the deceptive *policies*. Thus, the public, consulted in advance, might agree that, under certain circumstances, it would be appropriate for the government to deceive it.

It is ultimately, of course, an empirical proposition as to whether the government could satisfy these criteria for the moral justification of deception concerning the HIV epidemic. Given the present climate of eroding trust in the federal government, however, the probability of securing such a moral justification appears very, very small.

CONCLUSIONS

By making misleading statements which give some measure of false reassurance about the danger of HIV infection and AIDS, the majority of the AIDS information brochures reinforce the nation's avoidance of thinking about the epidemic and denial of its seriousness. There is no evidence that the high degree of similarity in the misleading statements of many brochures is the product of conscious conspiracy among officials of state health departments and federal agencies. It does appear probable, however—and understandable—that staff members of state health departments, the CDC, and other federal agencies have been influenced by the Reagan and Bush administrations' obvious desire to portray the epidemic as a minor concern which would have no impact on the majority of Americans.

The unfortunate consequence of this pervasive pattern of avoidance and denial within the federal and many state governments is that neither the public nor the political leaders have a clear sense of the epidemic, much less a realistic plan of action. Nowhere is this more strikingly demonstrated than in the illogical retention of the diagnostic term "AIDS" rather than the adoption of the scientifically correct term "HIV disease," which should be diagnosed when HIV infection is first determined. The majority of the AIDS information brochures deepen the confusion over the concept of HIV disease by failing to explain that HIV infection is believed always or virtually always to result eventually in "AIDS," which is simply the term given to the terminal stage of HIV disease.

The continued reliance upon an illogical diagnostic category is dangerous because it obscures the scope of the epidemic for both political leaders and ordinary citizens alike. The scope of the epidemic is not revealed accurately by the roughly one-quarter million people in the U.S. now living with "AIDS" but by the one-to-two million people now living with HIV disease. The National Parents' Council on AIDS reaffirms its recommendation that the diagnosis of "AIDS" be immediately discontinued and that the diagnosis of HIV disease be adopted for all who are infected with HIV.

The potentially destructive impact exerted by systematically misleading statements in the majority of the brochures raises a broader concern about the influence of governmental agencies on the flow of information regarding the HIV epidemic and other public health issues. Are there perhaps other, less visible, ways in which governmental manipulation of public health information occurs? Must we worry that wholesale suppression of information may have happened because of the apprehension of political leaders? Of the estimated 19,000 documents classified as secret each day by officials of federal agencies, must we be concerned that some contain important information about the HIV epidemic?

While it is clear that governments frequently practice deception and secrecy with the justification that the public would become dangerously emotional and irrational if fully informed, there is no evidence that the public would in fact behave in that way. Rather, a fully-informed public, confident in the integrity of its government, will be more courageous and resourceful in coping with catastrophe than one from which its government keeps secrets.

With these concerns in mind, the National Parents' Council on AIDS offers several recommendations regarding both the improvement of AIDS information brochures, and the broader issues of public access to information about the epidemic.

RECOMMENDATIONS ABOUT
AIDS INFORMATION BROCHURES

1. Both governmental and nongovernmental organizations should evaluate HIV/AIDS literature periodically in order to ensure that it is scientifically accurate and free from political bias. In particular, the four characteristics of the present medical model of AIDS reviewed in this study should be included in every publicly distributed brochure until such time as they may be replaced by advances in the model. There is no excuse for the extreme variation in quality of information among the brochures. A resident of one state should not receive information about HIV disease that is markedly inferior to that received by citizens of other states.

2. A few states and other agencies have produced outstanding AIDS information brochures; they should be emulated widely. It is not necessary for every state to write its own brochure to convey information about the HIV epidemic, although, of course, the states may need to append information about services specific to the states.

3. Special attention should be given to the deletion of out-of-date literature from the supplies available to the public. Many state departments of health and other agencies continue to distribute brochures which were once satisfactory but are now obsolete. While some older brochures are of high quality, there is a strong overall relationship between quality of information and recency of publication.

RECOMMENDATIONS CONCERNING BROADER ISSUES
OF PUBLIC ACCESS TO INFORMATION

1. The President and the Secretary of Health and Human Services should publicly declare, and then carry out, a policy of free and full disclosure of information concerning all aspects of the HIV epidemic.

2. The President should declare that the classification of HIV information as secret will not be permitted. If classification of such documents has occurred, that fact should be acknowledged and the affected documents made public.
3. The President and the Secretary of Health and Human Services should publicly declare, and then act accordingly, that no policy of prior review, editing, censorship, or delay in reporting of scientific or other information about the HIV epidemic or any other public health concern will be imposed upon any federal or nongovernmental agency, nor upon any individual.

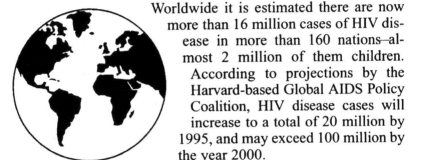 Worldwide it is estimated there are now more than 16 million cases of HIV disease in more than 160 nations—almost 2 million of them children. According to projections by the Harvard-based Global AIDS Policy Coalition, HIV disease cases will increase to a total of 20 million by 1995, and may exceed 100 million by the year 2000.

Policy Recommendation Number One:

It is now accepted by virtually all medical researchers that infection with HIV initiates a continuous, slowly-developing disease with a terminal phase characterized by what we now call AIDS. We conclude it is no longer rational to consider HIV infection and AIDS as separate categories. Therefore the National Parents' Council on AIDS urges immediate adoption of the following recommendation by the Centers for Disease Control and all other agencies and individuals dealing with the HIV epidemic:

Infection with HIV should be considered evidence of a single illness, called *HIV disease,* and the diagnoses of AIDS and ARC (AIDS-Related Complex) should be immediately discontinued.

We believe it is imperative that the recommended change in nomenclature be adopted at once in order not to obscure further the magnitude of the epidemic. Under the current case definition, there are now about 150,000 living persons with the AIDS diagnosis, but the reality is that there are an estimated one to two million people with *HIV disease,* all or virtually all of whom, it is believed, will eventually die should more effective treatments not be developed.

–National Parents' Council on AIDS

The Six Highest-Ranked Brochures

For the general public, regardless of educational level:
Red Cross–*"HIV Infection And AIDS'*

For readers educated in the academic upper half of high schools and/or in college:
Delaware–*"AIDS: Know The Facts And Be Safe"*
Michigan–*"AIDS And Everyone"*
Tennessee–*"AIDS And Sex: What You Should Know"*

For readers educated in the academic upper half of colleges:
American Council On Science And Health–
"Answers About AIDS"
American College Health Association–
"HIV Infection And AIDS"

ABOUT THE NATIONAL PARENTS' COUNCIL ON AIDS

The National Parents' Council on AIDS was formed in 1988 as a citizens' response to the unprecedented global health crisis of the HIV epidemic. The purpose of the NPCA is to help the nation define and work toward an effective response to the epidemic. The NPCA is not a support group for parents whose children have AIDS–that function is addressed effectively by other organizations. Rather, the NPCA represents the concerns of all parents–and all those who feel a parental responsibility for the young, whether or not they are biological parents.

The National Parents' Council on AIDS is concerned broadly with education and public policy regarding all aspects of the HIV epidemic, not just those pertaining to children, for the welfare of children cannot be addressed meaningfully in isolation, but only by addressing the ways in which the epidemic affects all citizens.

The activities and programs of the NPCA include:

- helping parents and other citizens acknowledge their personal responsibility for deciding upon and carrying out constructive responses to the HIV crisis;
- providing information to NPCA members and to the public concerning the actions of federal and state governments regarding the HIV epidemic and AIDS:
- serving as a research resource to, and consulting with, the federal and state governments and their agencies concerning more effective responses to the HIV crisis;
- publishing the *NPCA Quarterly Bulletin*, which reports broadly on matters of education and public policy regarding the HIV epidemic;
- developing syllabuses for educational programs concerning the HIV epidemic;
- sponsoring lectures on such topics as "What Should Be Our National Policy on HIV Disease?", "The Responsibilities of Fathers in the Age of AIDS," "The Role of Churches in the National Response to HIV Disease," and "Helping Children Understand HIV Disease."

Please feel free to contact the National Council on HIV-Disease at:

National Council on HIV-Disease
P.O. Box 66966
Phoenix, AZ 85082

The Social Construction
of Target Populations
and the Transformation
of Prison-Based AIDS Policy:
A Descriptive Case Study

Nancy Lynne Hogan, PhD

Morehead State University

SUMMARY. When interpreting policy changes, it is important to understand the social constructions of those whom the policy affects. Policy Design Perspective by Schneider and Ingram (1993) concentrates on the construction of "agents" and "targets" in an attempt to comprehend policy formation and transformation. The following descriptive case study uses this design to assess the evolution of one prison's AIDS policy. This institution's HIV/AIDS policy originally was quite restrictive in nature, but the changing perceptions of the agents and targets allowed a more humanistic approach to emerge in

Nancy Lynne Hogan is Assistant Professor in the Department of Sociology, Social Work, and Criminology at Morehead State University. Her background includes 13 years in corrections with five years specifically devoted to HIV/AIDS issues. Presently, she is continuing her research interests in corrections by focusing on correctional officers and the use of force.

Correspondence may be addressed: Department of Sociology, 318 Rader Hall, Morehead State University, Morehead, KY 40351 [E-mail: n.hogan@morehead-st.edu].

[Haworth co-indexing entry note]: "The Social Construction of Target Populations and the Transformation of Prison-Based AIDS Policy: A Descriptive Case Study." Hogan, Nancy Lynne. Co-published simultaneously in *Journal of Homosexuality* (The Haworth Press, Inc.) Vol. 32, No. 3/4, 1997, pp. 77-114; and: *Activism and Marginalization in the AIDS Crisis* (ed: Michael A. Hallett) The Haworth Press, Inc., 1997, pp. 77-114; and: *Activism and Marginalization in the AIDS Crisis* (ed: Michael A. Hallett) Harrington Park Press, an imprint of The Haworth Press, Inc., 1997, pp. 77-114. Single or multiple copies of this article are available for a fee from The Haworth Document Delivery Service [1-800-342-9678, 9:00 a.m. - 5:00 p.m. (EST). E-mail address: get info@haworth.com].

the handling of HIV-positive inmates. *[Article copies available for a fee from The Haworth Document Delivery Service: 1-800-342-9678. E-mail address: getinfo@haworth.com]*

One night in 1985, a small eastern county prison was introduced to the AIDS crisis while handling routine commitments. During the evening, two prisoners were brought into the institution for bad-check charges. In compliance with the initial booking procedure, the male and female defendants listed their hometown as a large metropolitan city. They were routinely asked if they were under the influence of alcohol or any drug. Both answered no. It was not until the conclusion of the booking process that the question dealing with medical problems arose. "Do you have ulcers, asthma, a heart condition, diabetes, or take any prescription medication?" Their answers changed the future course of action and policy guidelines for everyone involved at the facility. The female stated she took AZT for AIDS. The man, who was her boyfriend, stated that he thought he was also infected.

The booking officer along with those officers about to conduct the strip searches didn't know how to respond. AIDS was something that happened in big cities, not in an off-the-pace small town. No one really had any knowledge about the disease or any factual information about its transmission. Fear and panic were passed along the chain of command ending up with the warden. He instructed the captain to place the inmates in isolation until arrangements for admission at the local hospital could be planned. Orders were also given that anything touched by the inmates was to be bagged for incineration. Once the commitments were settled into isolation, the officers who had come in contact with the "disease" were permitted to leave their duty stations for showering. Each officer spent over 30 minutes in the hot shower, scrubbing themselves down to get the infection "off." Once showers were completed, a trustee was called to disinfect the locker room with bleach. All staff avoided the isolation cells as much as possible and when morning arrived, the medically isolated inmates were served breakfast on "throw away" Styrofoam.

As soon as the next shift took over, the assignment for hospital duty was announced. Fearful that they could somehow take the disease home and infect their families, the officers questioned man-

agement about transmission. Without adequate knowledge to pass on, those in charge defensively ordered individual officers to work at the hospital. Four officers refused to follow the direct order, which resulted in their 30-day suspension from work. Their non-compliance to management was viewed as a good decision by the majority of the correctional staff. Most officers were glad they were not put in the position of making such a choice. Those that accepted the hospital assignment did so reluctantly, more out of coercion and fear of management's punishment rather than their own choice. Upon transport to the hospital, the inmate's uniforms, bedding, and street clothes were incinerated.

After the inmates' admission to the hospital, the day was filled with networking and information-sharing. The administrator and his assistants called hospitals, the local health department, and the Centers for Disease Control in order to ascertain what AIDS was. At the same time, strategic planning was done within the criminal justice system to coordinate the outcome of the infected inmates' cases.

Unfortunately, the fear had already formed a strong foothold. The new "knowledge" provided by the administration about transmission and infection was met with powerful resistance by the line employees. Officers talked among themselves, questioning whether or not this new information was valid based on the initial managerial commands. "Why did management order us to burn the clothes; why were the inmates sent to the hospital; and why are the administrators working so hard to get the new admissions released as fast as possible?"

The infected inmates' stay was brief. Prior to release, the counselors were assigned to purchase new clothing to replace what was burned. Talking with the inmates via telephone, sizes and necessary items were determined. When the counselors brought the new clothes to the hospital, they were afraid to enter the inmates' rooms which were marked with brightly colored signs stating "Blood and Body Fluid Precautions." In order to avoid personal contact with the HIV-positive inmates, the newly purchased clothing was handed over to the correctional officer on duty. Charges were then dismissed and the "infected prisoners" were set free. The only condition of release was that they never return to the area.

This narrative provides a glimpse at the atmosphere in which most prison-based HIV/AIDS policies were developed and later transformed as a result of internal shifts in the social construction of seropositive inmates by correctional officers. At the beginning, lack of actual knowledge about the disease and an overabundance of fear served as the motivating forces behind policy formation. Tragically absent from the picture was the concern over whom the policy was to affect—the HIV-positive inmate. Powerless, the "infected" inmates were subjected to policies that were quite restrictive in order to alleviate employee and inmate population fear. These repressive directives were encouraged and supported by political leaders who voiced society's disdain toward criminally deviant groups.

The following essay will explore the evolution of HIV/AIDS policy within the above correctional setting. Through the use of participant observation, focus will be placed on general policy choices and the specific decision-making processes. It will be observed that the HIV-positive inmates' medical and emotional issues were not a primary consideration. Rather, a goal of AIDS correctional policy has been the maintenance of stability between the line personnel and the general inmate population. Organizational concerns have created a schism between HIV-positive inmates in relation to other inmates, the staff, and the administration. By viewing these inmates as different and deviant, restrictive and repressive policies have been supported.

Yet, the social constructions of people can be altered (Aiken & Musheno, 1994). The beginning of this transformation was seen in the interim years and continues today. It is hoped that by tracing the history of one policy's progression, other administrators will be encouraged to place the HIV-positive inmates' interests at the center of policy while giving them a voice in shaping future AIDS policy direction. To assess policy decisions, a theoretical framework developed by Schneider and Ingram (1993) that concentrates on the social construction of the targets of policy will be used to uncover the position that HIV-positive inmates have occupied within the correctional setting.

POLICY FORMATION AND THE SOCIAL CONSTRUCTION OF TARGETS

There are many approaches to formulating and evaluating public policy. Different theories see distinctive roles for policy and use different methods in ascertaining improved performance. Policy Design Perspective is unique as it incorporates the importance of human nature and its effects on policy formation as well as recognizing that a policy can reflect different theories at different times (Schneider & Ingram, 1994). The policy design paradigm is taken a step further by Schneider and Ingram, who explore the social constructions of "agents" and "targets" in relation to outcomes or goals (Schneider & Ingram, 1993). Through an analysis of the agents (those who implement the policy) and its "targets" (those at whom the policy is directed), a more complete understanding is formed about the nature of policy, its goals, and its outcomes (Schneider & Ingram, 1990b).

Concentration is placed on the social construction of the targets who are "those persons or groups which are expected to comply with the policy directives or who are offered policy opportunities" (Ingram & Schneider, 1991a, p. 334). The targets are viewed either positively or negatively, depending on their social construction within society. Political power, whether strong or weak, is also a focal point of a policy design. Power translates into the opportunity to get issues of concern on the political agenda. Those with strong political power are able to advance their own needs, which transposes into an overabundance of benefits while, at the same time, it creates an overabundance of burdens for negatively constructed, powerless groups.

Each policy design varies in the application of tools, rules, and assumptions which are applied differently depending on the social construction of the targets. Policy *tools* "are the devices used by elected or agency officials to provide motivation for the agents or target populations to carry out policy purposes" (Ingram & Schneider, 1991a, p. 337). Different types of tools are used to ensure compliance with a policy but vary depending on the agent's or target's construction. Authority tools assume targets will do as they are told to do and use a variety of motivators to ensure compliance. These can range from voluntary actions to use of force. Incentive tools "rely on tangible payoffs" to ensure compliance using monetary inducements, charges, sanctions, or force to counter resistance (Schneider & Ingram, 1990a, p. 515). Capacity tools provide information or training to carry out the policy while symbolic and hortatory tools assume that "people are motivated from within and decide whether or not to take policy-related actions on the basis of their beliefs and values" (Schneider & Ingram, 1990a, p. 519).

Rules "determine procedures, such as timing, evaluation requirements, and conditions for participation" (Ingram & Schneider, 1991b, p. 72) while "*theories* or *assumptions* explain why the tools and rules are expected to produce the intended behavior, and how the behavior is linked to the desired objectives" (Ingram & Schneider, 1991b, p. 72).

Schneider and Ingram's policy design model provides four categories for understanding the distribution of policy benefits and burdens. They are the advantaged, the contenders, the dependents, and the deviants (see Figure 1, p. 108).

The *advantaged* group is viewed positively and has strong political power. Policy, no matter how worded, will provide a benefit for this group. They have the most access to political leaders in order to meet their own needs and are able to voice their concerns within the political arena. They are viewed by society as deserving and intelligent; policy tools will emphasize "capacity building, inducements, and techniques that enable the target population to learn about the results of its behavior and take appropriate actions on a voluntary basis" (Schneider & Ingram, 1993, p. 339). Benefits from the policy will be oversubscribed while burdens will be undersubscribed (Schneider & Ingram, 1993).

Contenders also have strong political power but have been constructed negatively by society. This group has enough influence to affect the political agenda in order to advance their position. When policy benefits are given to contenders, they are often masked while burdens are overstated even though their overall impact is limited (Schneider & Ingram, 1993).

Dependents are looked at positively by society but are relatively powerless in affecting policy direction. Benefits for this group are very rule oriented, requiring stringent proof of eligibility. Often-times, funding is inadequate to meet the goals of policy directed at this group. Benefits, therefore, are undersubscribed (Schneider & Ingram, 1993).

Deviants emerge as the last category. Powerless, deviants are negatively constructed by society and are seen as the least deserving of benefits. When gains are made, political leaders justify their actions by framing the benefits as unavoidable (Schneider & Ingram, 1993). Burdens are oversubscribed and compliance to policy is ensured through coercion, punishment, or force.

These categories are not stagnant. Movement readily occurs when support and power are altered. Support can include financial resources and/or backing by more powerful groups or leaders. The transformation of a particular social construction can also occur by the organizing within a specific group or the restructuring of their present image. This can create wider sponsorship and alliances by closing the social distance between the groups' needs and those found in the larger population (Aiken & Musheno, 1994).

Public policy on AIDS reflects these categories in the presenta-tion of the disease as well as uncovering the beneficiaries of fund-ing. AIDS, in general, has been constructed negatively by classify-ing it as a "sexually transmitted disease rather than as a viral disease" (Donovan, 1994, p. 9). Descriptions of the disease and those infected often involve metaphors that have deeper meanings (Ross, 1988). For example, the media presentation of HIV-positive persons has created a dichotomy between innocent victims and those responsible for their own infection (Ross, 1988). This has allowed certain HIV-positive individuals to be negatively constructed and to be blamed for their plight.

In using the Schneider and Ingram model, those advantaged by AIDS public policy have been researchers, the medical field, the Centers for Disease Control, and health departments (Donovan, 1994, p. 5). The contenders have been politically strong AIDS advo-cates, including the Lambda Legal Defense Fund, Act Out, and the ACLU.[1] Strong political power also has allowed many members of the gay population to reconstruct their image away from a deviant construction in order to advance their agenda (Aiken & Musheno, 1994). Yet, Schneider and Ingram (1993) note that many times benefits gained by contenders have been outwardly presented as achievements for more positively constructed target groups.[2] The dependents are reflected in the population which has been referred to as the "innocent victims" of this disease. Children, hemophiliacs,[3] and women unknowingly infected by their partners account for a positive construction in society but lack political power to promote their concerns. Finally, the deviant category is made up of those already morally condemned by society. Drug users, prostitutes, people of color, and criminals are negatively constructed and are envisioned as less deserving of benefits while being held accountable for their own fates (Aiken & Musheno, 1994; Donovan, 1994; Hogan, 1994; Schneider & Ingram, 1993). Members of the gay population who also share one of these constructions have not risen to the contender role. The commonality reflected in the deviant category includes lower socio-economic status, lack of representation in the policy arena, and the powerlessness to change positions.

THE CONSTRUCTION OF POPULATIONS IN THE CORRECTIONAL SETTING

Schneider and Ingram's (1993) model can also effectively explain policy on a micro-level. Over the years, correctional AIDS policies have been established which provide benefits to the advantaged groups while overburdening the deviant groups. In the prison environment, the four categories of populations also exist. At the beginning of AIDS policy formation, the correctional staff emerged as the advantaged group; the noninfected inmates occupied the dependent group; and the HIV-positive inmates were placed in the deviant classification. The contender group was primarily represented by outside activist groups and a few advocates within the prison system.[4] Each area will be looked at in more detail.

Advantaged Group–The Staff

Normally, within the institutional setting, administrators are advantaged and create policy which reflects their own interests.

Budgetary concerns, liability, the maintenance of prison stability, and career advancement predominate policy direction. Generally, there have been deep fissures between management and line personnel (Jurik & Musheno, 1986). Most officers and staff have been voiceless in affecting policy direction of daily rules and procedures. The AIDS epidemic created an atmosphere that pushed these adversarial forces together. Administrators tend to side with staff concerns about HIV/AIDS and the possible intraprison transmission feared from routine contact. This has allowed the staff to emerge as the advantaged population in the development of AIDS correctional policies. Most restrictive policy arguments have always mentioned staff safety. This support translates into the oversubscription of benefits as predicted by Schneider and Ingram (Schneider & Ingram, 1993, p. 337).

The Contenders—Activists, Medical Staff, and Social Workers

At the beginning of correctional AIDS policy formation, contenders represented those who, by either compassion or increased knowledge, were less fearful of transmission. Within the system, medical personnel have always been in conflict with prison objectives. The goal of incarceration has been to segregate and punish offenders while the medical field's goal has been to provide comfort and care (Dubler & Sidel, 1991). This contradiction has created tension between the administrators and the medical staff, who were the first to question existing AIDS policies and began advocating for more leniency. Primarily, though, the contenders have been outside the criminal justice system. AIDS activist groups, inmate rights groups, and gay activist groups are responsible for advancing many of the issues that are of concern today.

The Dependents—Noninfected Inmates

The noninfected inmates, surprisingly, emerge as the dependent group. Ordinarily seen as deviant within the normal prison policy framework, fear of intraprison exposure has led this group to support the same restrictive policy requests as the officers. In fact, noninfected inmates became a driving force in the legal arena as well. Lawsuits on behalf of the general prison population have been filed supporting the very issues that correctional staff want addressed.[5] Most lawsuits have concentrated on issues of mass testing and segregation (Feigley v. Fulcomer, Glick v. Henderson, Jarrett v. Faulkner).[6]

In the Schneider and Ingram model, "officials want to appear to be aligned with their [dependents'] interests; but their lack of political power makes it difficult to direct resources toward them" (Schneider & Ingram, 1993, p. 338). Informally, inmates are encouraged to file lawsuits which benefit administrative goals. Yet, AIDS correctional policies provide little benefit to the noninfected population, while at the same time they create burdens by adding procedures. The general inmate population, for the most part, has supported the beliefs of the advantaged staff and has not objected to the more restrictive and invasive rules that affect their freedom within the institution.

The Deviants–HIV-Positive Inmates

Reflecting society's reaction to AIDS, the target group has been bitterly opposed. Panic and fear have been fundamental in working against any benefits being provided to this group. When benefits, such as increased medical attention, do occur, it is often an unavoidable consequence of rationales being used for restrictive policies. The concerns of the HIV-positive inmates were not addressed in the early years of correctional AIDS policy, and even today most policies are still being designed to address the needs of the advantaged and the dependent groups rather than the deviant groups.

In order to understand the emergent roles of each of these categories in AIDS correctional policy, the following descriptive case study will examine one prison's AIDS policy formation. The chronological development and revisions have been divided into three groups: 1985-1987, 1988-1990, and 1992 to the present. In each time period, general information available to all correctional institutions will be provided along with the specific areas of concern. Although the nature of this study is limited to one county prison, it allows a glimpse at correctional policy formation and the rationales behind the decision-making process. Schneider and Ingram's model will be utilized to uncover how policy benefits and burdens were assigned within the institution. It will be shown that any gain made for the deviant HIV-positive inmates always provided a hidden benefit for the advantaged group.

THE FORMATION OF RESTRICTIVE POLICIES: 1985-1987

In the mid-eighties, very few institutions had encountered HIV-positive inmates and had not proactively developed HIV/AIDS policy. General knowledge released to the public presented the infection as being concentrated in specific populations: the gay population, intravenous drug users, and promiscuous women. Also, a disproportionate amount of those becoming infected appeared to be lower-class minorities. These groups reflected the prison population which generated "concern that prisons might become sink holes for this modern pestilence" (Martin & Zimmerman, 1990, p. 330).

For prisons, the attention was focused on intravenous drug users (Vlahov, 1990; Hammett & Moini, 1990; Olivero & Roberts, 1989; Blumberg, 1989; Hammett, 1986a, 1986b) and prostitutes (Darrow, 1990; Leonard & Thistlethwaite, 1990; Cohen, Alexander, & Wofsy, 1988). The potential spread of HIV infection within the prison was also a major concern. Homosexual contact, sharing needles, tattooing (Martin & Zimmerman, 1990; Blumberg, 1989), rape (Hammett & Moini, 1990), biting, and spitting (Blumberg & Langston, 1991) were viewed as possible transmission routes.

Fear and anxiety inspired most correctional agencies to begin formulating rules and procedures to deal with the prospect of housing HIV-positive inmates. In most institutions, three interlacing goals shaped the policy's content. They were security, liability, and cost-effectiveness. By briefly discussing each, a better understanding will emerge of how these goals molded final policy decisions.

The major objective of any correctional facility was and is security. In order for this to be accomplished, there must be stability between the staff and the inmate population. Frightened by the prospect of exposure to an incurable virus, guards and inmates threatened to upset this delicate balance. In 1986, The National Institute of Justice published the first comprehensive guide on AIDS issues for corrections. It advised that "correctional administrators formulate policies that allowed them to manage their institutions effectively, while dealing with a serious health problem that may cause fear among the staff and inmates" (Hammett, 1986a). Yet, reports of guards refusing to work with infected inmates, ignoring inmate requests, and failing to fulfill daily routines presented a major concern (Olivero, 1989). The noninfected inmates also reacted by threatening to harm HIV-positive inmates if they were placed in general population. Accounts of beatings and threats of arson circulated among administrators (Olivero, 1989). Thus, policy makers kept in mind directives which would maintain control over the inmate population and the correctional staff as well.

Liability was also a concern. Several lawsuits had already been filed dealing with issues of medical care, confidentiality, and housing status. It was recommended that these issues be carefully addressed in preparing policy (Hammett, 1986b). Yet, to most administrators, liability meant developing a policy which preserved the safety of the staff and the general inmate population. It was assumed that lawsuits could be prevented by focusing on limiting possible intraprison transmission.

Finally, cost played a significant role in policy development. Overcrowding had already strained most correctional funds without the added expense for HIV testing. If funding was added for identification purposes, positive test results would require some provision of medical care for those infected. This could prove costly. In 1986, the initial antibody blood test (ELISA) ranged from $5 to $10 (Hammett, 1986b, p. 36). If positive, a much more detailed and expensive confirmatory test was needed. The Western Blot confirmatory test averaged about $75 (Hammett, 1986b, p. 36). Also, the Centers for Disease Control recommended follow-up testing to cover the "window period."[7] These expenses were for the identification of HIV-positive inmates only. Once they were distinguished as HIV-positive, providing minimal care, such as regular blood work and checkups with specialists, could quickly drain medical funds. In the mid-eighties, medication alone could cost up to $10,000 per year (Hammett, 1988, p. 82).[8]

Thus, security, liability, and cost-effectiveness played a major role in individual correctional facility decisions concerning the formation of HIV policy. Issues of policy concern that were focused on included: HIV testing, confidentiality of test results, housing assignments of HIV-positive inmates, and their participation in general inmate activities. These policy areas and the different options open to correctional facilities will be presented below.

Testing

Testing was brought to the forefront of policy for the purpose of identification of those who were seropositive.[9] In order to identify the HIV carriers, mandatory screening of all inmates was widely supported. Proponents provided a variety of reasons why mandatory screening was preferred. One rationale stated that it would "serve to allay fears of AIDS within correctional institutions more effectively than any education program" (Hammett, 1986b, p. 36). Other reasons cited identification of HIV-positive inmates for education programs, prevention, medical care, and the use of precautionary measures by the staff (Carroll, 1992; Blumberg, 1989; Hammett, 1988, 1986a). Opponents to this stance stated that there was no proof of higher rates of transmission in prisons and that mass screening could possibly lead to increased fear and segregation of the infected inmate (Hammett, 1986a, 1986b). Opponents preferred policies of education and prevention methods.

Mandatory testing, though, was widely supported by society. Bayer points out that in 1987, 88% of Americans supported mass screening of federal prisoners (Bayer, 1989, p. 166). This was answered by President Reagan in a May 1987 speech in which he advocated mandatory testing of federal prisoners despite the objection of the surgeon general (Bayer, 1989, p. 164). Even the American Medical Association supported this recommendation (JAMA Board of Trustees, 1987).

Although several correctional systems decided to mass screen, most facilities chose other alternatives. A popular method was high-risk testing. Rather than screen all inmates, high-risk testing focused on certain known behaviors of inmates. Other choices included testing upon clinical indications, voluntary testing, or deliberately not testing (Hammett, 1986b). Hammett indicates that in 1986, four state systems required mass screening while most jurisdictions chose more limited testing (Hammett, 1986a).[10]

County Prison Response

Pressure from the media and the political arena persuaded many institutions to begin developing a policy. Despite the initial encounter with two HIV-positive commitments, two years passed before the county facility felt an urgency to formulate a policy. Concerned about security and liability, choices about testing were not easy. Any decision of institution-initiated testing would prove expensive, but the officers and inmates were quite vocal in demanding identification of infected inmates. This paralleled the political climate of the time, which lent support to testing by providing funds. In an effort to employ some type of cost-effectiveness, like many other facilities, high-risk behavior testing was adopted. Upon admission to the facility, classification focused on certain known behaviors conducive to infection. The policy stated:

> Targeted groups include intravenous drug users, homosexual or bisexual men, lesbian or bisexual women, high risk pregnant women, male and female prostitutes, hemophiliacs, and any inmate returned or brought to the facility from another institution that is deemed to be high risk. (County Prison, 1987, p. 7)

HIV testing was targeted at new commitments, but a primary concern was infection from fighting, biting, spitting, tattooing, needle sharing, and shaving. Inclusive in the policy was a section to cover these issues:

> Any individuals [inmates] involved in incidents where blood and body fluids are exchanged should be immediately tested to determine whether or not anyone was seropositive at the time of the incident. (County Prison, 1987, p. 7)

Choices for testing illustrate the power differentials and positions that agents and targets occupy in policy formation. Agents, lacking direct knowledge about HIV/AIDS, turned to outside agencies to provide information and guidance in the creation of policy directives. This pushed the development of the policy in a restrictive direction. Targets were "criminals" who were further denounced by society as "HIV carriers." No sympathy was given to this double-stigmatized group, and medical benefits were vividly lacking in the stated rationales. Yet targets are oversubscribed with burdens (Schneider & Ingram, 1993). Funds were readily available for testing procedures to identify those infected. Many of the concerns voiced by the advantaged group, the officers, were carefully considered and incorporated into the new procedures. The dependents, noninfected inmates, were pleased with the protocol, despite many having to submit to testing. The targets, though, were never represented as players in the policy formation.

Confidentiality

The area of most concern regarding restrictive policies was confidentiality of the medical results. Proponents argued that correctional staff, due to daily contact with inmates, had a "need to know" in order to prevent possible contact with blood and body fluids. Disclosure to the staff was deemed a legal and moral responsibility to protect staff and inmates which was thought to take precedence over the HIV-positive inmates' right to privacy (Hammett, 1986b, p. 55). Critics of this stance argued for strict policies where confidentiality was maintained in order to prevent "ostracism, threats, and possibly violent intimidation while in prison, and discrimination in employment, housing, and insurance availability after they are discharged" (Hammett, 1986b, p. 56). At this time, about one third of county and state systems disclosed names of HIV-positive inmates to correctional officers with over two thirds of the institutions disclosing HIV status to medical personnel (Hammett, 1986b).

County Prison Response

The correctional officers and staff wanted to know the names of those infected in order to take precautions against possible exposure. Unconfirmed media reports questioned transmission routes already presented.[11] The dependent inmates also wanted the staff to know in order that infected inmates could be kept out of general population. Targets were to be feared, and although an attempt to consider their position was mentioned, the policy reflected the staff and inmate concerns:

> All inmates have the right to privacy and individual human dignity. Due to the adverse publicity of AIDS, the staff must pay special attention to the confidentiality of the inmates' diagnosis. Any communication within the institution should be kept to a minimum and precautions should be taken not to discuss an inmate's diagnosis where it can be overheard by other inmates. At no time should any staff member broadcast a patient's diagnosis, medical condition, sexual orientation, or personal habits to anyone not associated with this institution. The exceptions are as follows: (1) any extra-institutional staff (police, constables, sheriffs, paramedics, etc.) who have contact with the inmate shall be notified prior to contact, [and] (2) transfers between correctional institutions shall have updated medical summaries including HIV infection. (County Prison, 1987, p. 8)[12]

Housing Assignments

Once seropositivity was determined, housing became a controversial issue. Segregation from general population was promoted in order to prevent inmate violence as well as possible transmission through sexual activity, needle sharing, or tattooing (Blumberg, 1989; Olivero, 1989; Hammett, 1986a).[13] Opponents argued that segregation undermines the public health message that AIDS is not spread through casual contact (Blumberg, 1989, p. 6).

Choices of administrators were isolation, separation in a designated unit or medical block, hospitalization, or general population (Hammett, 1986b). Yet, HIV testing set out to identify those who were infected in order to "protect the staff and inmates." This rationale led to restrictive housing choices—a choice other than mainstream population.

County Prison Response

The county prison believed that liability could be reduced by taking steps to prevent possible exposure to staff and inmates. The policy choice was the most restrictive housing assignment with the least amount of freedom:

> Once it is determined that an inmate is in a high-risk category and he/she is to be tested, the inmate is to be administratively isolated or double-locked until the results are known. Housing for seropositive inmates will be handled on a case by case basis and will be determined by the counseling staff and security staff. Such cases will depend on overcrowded conditions, security, and medical considerations. Whenever possible, isolation will be used. (County Prison, 1987, p. 7)

Housing assignments again favored the staff and noninfected inmates. The primary thought was to separate those who could prove deadly. No genuine consideration was given to inmates who were just informed of seropositivity, their mental and emotional needs, and their need for comfort and support. Although medical care was part of the picture, housing assignments were primarily chosen by administrators for what they thought to be "infection control."

Participation in Activities

In institutions where segregation of HIV-infected inmates existed, participation in activities was also addressed. Fear of possible transmission or prison disorder prompted most administrators to limit HIV-positive inmates' participation in gym, educational programs, law library, visiting, church services, and work release. Opponents stated that this was discriminatory because it prevented many inmates from gaining good time credits needed for early release (Blumberg, 1989). The courts required that inmates participate in certain activities such as gym, law library, and visiting. In order to meet this requirement, separate times were established to prevent the mixing of the infected with the noninfected.

County Prison Response

The county prison chose "separate but equal" in its policy directives. Within each guideline, the rationale was explicitly stated:

Food Service: Due to the correctional setting, it is advised that no inmate suspected or diagnosed as seropositive be allowed in the kitchen area. Due to uncleanliness or vengeful tactics, an inmate could put body fluids in the prepared food.

Visiting: Separate visiting times will be scheduled due to the presence of other inmates who may be fearful or cause the infected inmate humiliation in front of his visitors.

Gym procedures: Cuts or body contact are always a possibility during any supervised gym period. Therefore, the seropositive inmates will receive gym time separate from general population to reduce any possible accident of this nature.

General activities: Participation in GED, AA or drug treatment presents no risk to the staff or general population in an ideal situation where confidentiality can be maintained. In order to protect them from general population, they will not be allowed to attend. The prison will make every attempt to provide the individual counseling on a one-to-one basis in areas of need.

Law library: Seropositive inmates will be allowed to use our law library at a separate time if requested [cites constitutional right to access].

Church services: Although there is no risk in allowing a seropositive inmate to participate in church service, it must be taken into consideration the reaction from inmates in general population and the likely result would be disruption in prison order. (County Prison, 1987, pp. 11-12)

These policies supported the dependent-general population inmates who wanted no contact with HIV-positive inmates. Officers also favored this position as it reduced their daily contact with those infected.

IMPLEMENTATION OF RESTRICTIVE POLICIES

The advantaged population was quite pleased with the strict policy adopted. Staff were issued a variety of equipment to prevent possible infection including CPR masks, latex gloves, and protective body gear. Special cleaning solutions and bleach were purchased to handle any blood and body fluid spills. Even red infectious garbage bags were ordered to separate AIDS-infected garbage from the general trash. Cooperation was gained through the use of capacity tools which assumed that information would inspire changed behavior (Schneider & Ingram, 1993). Rules involved paid mandatory training sessions which were held to inform the staff about HIV/AIDS and to discuss the new procedures. All precautions were taken to the extreme in order to protect the staff. Even intraprison transport required the use of two officers, one required to carry a nightstick, and the use of handcuffs on the HIV-positive inmate. Questions about the disease were answered, and assurance from the warden was given that the officers' interests were the chief concern of the administration. Schneider and Ingram (1993) note that policy makers are quite supportive of the powerful, positively constructed groups. Their issues are held and responded to in a framework that is almost always advantageous.

The dependents were also quite satisfied with the strict procedures. Many new commitments fell into a high-risk category and were required to be tested. Despite the inconvenience, the noninfected inmates were guaranteed their own protection and safety.

The contenders within the system had yet to emerge. Although medical personnel questioned some of the directives, no one at this early stage was really knowledgeable enough to make a counterclaim against the instituted guidelines. In more progressive jurisdictions, testing, housing, and treatment issues of HIV-infected inmates were a focal point of controversy. The ACLU and the Lambda Legal Defense Fund showed interest in these issues, but most lawsuits on behalf of HIV-positive inmates were futile due to the courts' deference to stated penological interests (Gregware, 1994).

In short, the targets were just that—targets. They remained faceless, unidentified carriers of a highly feared disease. No further encounters with any seropositive inmate had since occurred at the prison and this invisibility allowed policy guidelines to be constructed without considering the adverse effects created by isolation, ostracism, and fear.

The first few identified HIV-positive inmates were shocked and hurt by the treatment they received. Despite being known and liked by the correctional staff, they were not prepared for the outward hostility and fear presented by the workers. Many of the staff refused to answer their requests, spoke to them from a distance, and took all precautions when transporting them within the institution. This special treatment was quite noticeable to the other inmates and reinforced the anxiety which already plagued the institution.

The isolation cell itself was traumatic. Designed for punishment, these small rooms were not equipped with radios or TVs. Lighting was poor, making reading or letter writing difficult. Left alone, there was too much time to think about the disease and its impending doom. Being deprived normal daily "time fillers" such as participation in activities or even conversation with other inmates soon took its toll on the HIV-positive inmates leaving them depressed and emotionally distraught without comfort, support, or information to ease their fears.

Coercion was used to insure cooperation with the policy. Fearing longer incarceration, the HIV-positive inmates never resisted being handcuffed nor did they verbally complain about the many invasive procedures. They reluctantly accepted the segregation from general population and remained silent and respectful despite overhearing negative comments from the officers and the other inmates.

The daily routine for the targets served as a reminder of their status. Anything handed to them by the officers was done with latex gloves on. Everything the HIV-positive inmates touched was immediately disinfected with bleach.[14] Their food was served on disposable trays and any garbage from their cell was placed in red infectious bags. Even their uniforms and bed linens were washed separately in hot water and bleach.

The deviant targets had no voice in their treatment within the facility and they were powerless to affect its change. Even in the testing process itself, there was no choice. If an inmate deemed high risk refused to be HIV tested, a court order was issued requiring involuntary testing. Once it was explained that noncompliance resulted in the same outcome, most inmates "voluntarily" submitted.

Yet, without knowing it, their silence and cooperation provided the foundation for future policy changes and a more humanistic approach to HIV infection within the county prison.

THE INTERIM YEARS–1988-1990

The Schneider and Ingram model can be expanded to account for the alterations to any policy group's social construction. Cultural images are relative and evolve and fluctuate over time. Power, both financial and political, is not static and is interactive with emerging social constructions. Although the model does not expressly account for these shifts, it is evident that policies are adjusted and developed according to the needs of the agents and targets within a given era. This is reflected in the growth and transformation of AIDS correctional policy in the interim years.

Most people in society did not have direct contact with the HIV-positive population and continued to support restrictive measures. Reflecting the tone set by society, political leaders called for quarantine, criminal sanctions, and mass testing in immigration, the armed forces, and marriage applications, which allowed the aura of fear to persist (Jones & Bishop, 1990; Hammett, 1988, p. 69). Public reaction influences much policy direction where officials try to avoid criticism (Schneider & Ingram, 1994).

Yet, in general, many correctional institutions were forced to deal with HIV-positive inmates which provided direct hands-on experience. Political pressure provided external motivation to continue restrictive measures, while internally, many prisons were encountering management problems with earlier policy choices. Coinciding with this growing tension was the medical field's increased knowledge about HIV/AIDS, research on risk and transmission, and court decisions which supported less restrictive measures.

If an AIDS policy had not been developed, most facilities began to feel political pressure to formulate one (Hammett, 1988, p. 70). Increased knowledge about AIDS aided policy makers in making many managerial decisions. The initial fear and anxiety of transmission was eased with the continual confirmation of blood to blood exposure, sexual contact, and perinatal contact and the dismissal of other modes such as mosquitoes, biting, and spitting.

The pattern of infection for those incarcerated with HIV was predominantly intravenous drug use.[15] Secondly, most systems adopted training for their staff in order to quell any apprehension about working with HIV-positive inmates (Hammett, 1988). Education and increased medical knowledge helped to change many systems' policies on testing and housing.

The expense of testing was phenomenal. The political arena continued calling for mass screening in order to prevent transmission within the institution, yet, other than a few locations, most systems were finding low percentages of infected inmates (Hammett, 1989).[16] In fact, systems that performed voluntary testing found higher seropositivity, which proved to be more cost-effective (Hammett, 1989). Thus, earlier predictions were not validated that HIV infection within the prison population would reach epidemic proportions.

Intraprison transmission of HIV was also unconfirmed. Only a few studies had been conducted and had concluded that transmission within the institution was quite rare.[17] Also, despite officers' fear of transmission, no correctional officer or police officer had become seropositive from a work exposure (Hammett, 1989).[18] Within 3 years, the trend to mass screen slowed with the replacement of more cost-effective measures: voluntary testing and clinically indicated testing. By the end of 1990, 15 state systems and the Federal Bureau of Prisons mass screened. No county or city system's budget could cover this added expense.

Funds were needed, though, to maintain adequate medical care. The intravenous drug users appeared to be more susceptible to pneumocystis carinii, which required longer hospitalization (Hammett, 1989, p. 39). In-house care for those manifesting symptoms was quoted as costing between $10,000 and $50,000 per inmate, while community hospitalization was said to run between $15,000 and $150,000 per inmate (Hammett, 1988, p. 81). Although the price of AZT had been reduced considerably, the medical community was calling for its usage at a much earlier stage in order to prolong the quality of life (Takas & Hammett, 1989; World Health Communications, 1988).[19]

Housing assignments were altered and most systems decided against blanket segregation (Hammett, 1988). Many institutions began to segregate HIV-positive inmates who were symptomatic.[20]

From an administrators' point of view, mainstreaming asymptomatic HIV-positive inmates was needed because of serious overcrowding. Cell space was not available to house seropositive inmates separate from general population as segregation and isolation were needed for behavior problems. Still the Centers for Disease Control recommended special housing for ARC/AIDS inmates, and most penal systems complied (Hammett, 1988, p. 84). By the end of 1991, the trend changed to a "case by case" basis for housing decisions stating that "segregation or separation may be impractical and unfeasible" (Hammett & Moini, 1990, p. 8).

Medically, several changes in procedure occurred. In order to ascertain possible high-risk behavior, institutions began doing in-depth medical histories on inmates and providing more complete physical examinations (Hammett, 1988, p. 79). The CDC released guidelines that now included pre- and posttest counseling prior to anyone submitting to an HIV test and the re-emphasis on universal precautions in order to combat HIV infection as well as hepatitis and tuberculosis (MMWR, 1987). Increased knowledge on HIV allowed many medical departments to take an active role within the prison in discussing the course of action for the inmates.

Outside influence was provided by the judicial system. The courts had an active role in molding policy due to the inactivity of Congress, the President, or the Supreme Court (Jones & Bishop, 1990, p. 284). Lawsuits which were filed focused on five legal issues: "testing, confidentiality, segregation, adequacy of care, and charging and convicting prisoners with AIDS who attack correctional officers" (Belbot & del Carmen, 1991, p. 135). Despite no definitive answers, different district courts set a variety of guidelines. Most courts, though, favored the correctional position on policies, citing legitimate penological interest (Aiken & Musheno, 1994; Gregware, 1994; Burris, 1992; Belbot & del Carmen, 1991). Despite most rulings favoring corrections, administrators were highly concerned about the prevention of lawsuits and kept close watch on issues that would affect current policies.

Thus, in the interim, many correctional facilities within the region of the county prison that had an AIDS policy slowly made modifications in order to alleviate overcrowding and budget constraints.[21] Those facilities that did not have a written policy were politically encouraged to do so out of concern over liability. There was the added benefit to those beginning to develop procedures–they had the experiences of other facilities to make better choices. Also, most institutions no longer relied solely on outside agencies to provide needed information about AIDS. Specialists within the facility aided administrators in making more informed decisions in respect to corrections.

County Prison Response–The Changing Social Constructions

The county facility felt the political pressures and took note of the abundance of court cases. Publications to provide an update on legal issues were subscribed to, and modifications in the policy were made when necessary.

Additions to the first policy now included testing of Haitians and Central Africans (County Prison, 1988, p. 6). Also HIV testing was required for any inmate who wanted to be a trustee (1988, p. 12). Most changes, though, were the clarification of procedures and more precise instructions for administering CPR, infection prevention, and the clean-up of blood and body fluid spillages. In an effort to alleviate overcrowding, housing of HIV-positive inmates reflected a "case by case" determination. Housing assignments could involve the use of double-lock, medical isolation, or the continued use of punitive isolation.

During these incremental changes, however, the correctional staff still remained advantaged. Most changes occurred at their insistence. Two issues emerged to push for a change. First, the officers began to complain about the extra work load that was needed to comply with the strict policy. The requirement of two officers for transport within the prison quickly was reduced to one due to staffing problems. Handcuffs became burdensome, searching for latex gloves became tedious, and 15-minute visual checks were thought to be unnecessary.[22] Several incidents occurred when isolation housing was needed for a violent inmate and the HIV-positive inmate was the only reasonable choice to be relocated. Second, and more important, the HIV-positive inmates were nonviolent and cooperative. Most had been incarcerated in the past and got along well with the staff. Officers began bringing in magazines and giving their newspaper to the inmates in order to lessen their boredom. The initial policy had been designed to deal with HIV-positive inmates, not human beings who were known and liked. The realization of people being infected brought out compassion and sympathy. Now able to identify the faces of HIV-positive inmates, the advantaged group began to slowly change their hard-line stance and began pushing for more lenient policies.

The general population inmates were also changing positions. Living in a small city, most of the inmates knew each other. Those infected had friends and acquaintances within the system. Due to the high numbers of inmates who had participated in drug usage, sympathy was immediately given to their unlucky associates.[23] Few problems occurred when asymptomatic inmates were placed in situations where there was contact with other inmates, even when their diagnosis was well known on the street.

The biggest change during these years was the emergence of the contender group. The medical staff and HIV counselors became increasingly knowledgeable and readily voiced their concerns over policy decisions. The major motivator for the medical staff was the continuation of being certified by the American Medical Association. Few small county institutions held this honor, and in order to be recertified, the quality of care had to meet the Association's existing standards. Therefore, medical personnel advocated changes that were more humanistic and representative of the HIV-inmates' health interests. Outside the prison, the health department and the local AIDS council took an avid interest in the prison policy and became activists for reform. When more liberal changes were made, these outside agencies provided an added incentive with their acceptance of the policy direction.

The deviant target group finally began to develop a face. More than one HIV-positive inmate incarcerated became the norm which made it increasingly difficult to envision that AIDS would just go away. Although last on the list in terms of factors affecting the decision-making process, their cooperativeness allowed advocates to advance their concerns. Yet, policy alterations were not a direct result of this group. Still, their powerless position provided no voice in the policy direction unless it was voiced by the contenders or the advantaged group. Despite many "enlightened" options in the county prison policy, the targets still had their share of burdens.

Fear and anxiety still persisted among several staff members and this was reflected in their attitude towards those infected. The revised policy still allowed stricter measures as an option and a few officers insisted on handcuffs and/or gloves. These choices stood apart from the majority of officers, who preferred the use of general procedures. This constant contradiction of treatment created confusion among the HIV-positive inmates.

Behavior of the HIV-positive inmates was placed in the forefront and used as a tool for compliance. Advancements made in housing or programming could be quickly changed if the HIV-positive inmates' attitude or behavior was not deemed appropriate. This was especially difficult when certain officers still remained hostile. Those that could play the game the best were rewarded with being "treated like an inmate." Those that had difficulty dealing with incarceration and their disease remained ostracized and treated as deviants.

TODAY AND BEYOND

Today most correctional systems have gained control over policy direction on HIV and have incorporated a more expanded mission than seen in the past. When the epidemic first occurred, corrections was expected to prevent further transmission within the correctional institution (Hammett, 1986b). Today "an expanded mission has emerged for correctional policy to focus on HIV/AIDS education intervention which not only benefits the institution, but also benefits society as a whole" (Hogan, 1994, p. 220). The emphasis is now to educate the prison population who have been hard to reach through government funded prevention efforts (Hammett, Harrold, Gross, & Epstein, 1994; Hogan, 1994; Christensen, 1990; Porter, 1988; Turner, Miller, & Moses, 1989). Corrections, in general, has the ability to be the initiator of societal good through the education of inmates in order to prevent transmission outside the institution (Hogan, 1994). This has sparked a proactive effort to provide quality education within the institution. Currently, HIV education for inmates and staff training are provided in the federal prisons, almost all state systems, and over half of the county/city facilities (Hammett et al., 1994, pp. 32, 34).

Policies on HIV testing have remained stable since 1990 with no additional state or local systems adopting mass screening procedures (Hammett et al., 1994, p. 49). The reduction of fear due to intraprison transmission continues. No correctional officer has been infected in the workplace and transmission among inmates remains low (Hammett et al., 1994). Confidentiality also is being tightened with fewer than 20% of county/city and fewer than 12% of state systems informing correctional officers (Hammett et al., 1994, p. 55).

Overcrowding has continued to plague corrections, which has resulted in the further reduction of blanket segregation policies. Segregation and isolation continue to be abandoned in favor of case by case housing assignments. Only three state systems and three county/city systems permanently segregate asymptomatic inmates (Hammett et al., 1994, p. 59).

Medical care and the availability of medication continue to improve. By 1992, almost all systems offered AZT when clinically called for (Hammett et al., 1994 p. 70). Unfortunately, access to clinical trials seems to be a major stumbling block (Hammett et al., 1994, p. 70).

The legal climate still has offered no definitive course of action for corrections officials in cases involving confidentiality, segregation, mandatory testing, access to programs, and medical care. For the most part, corrections policy has still been upheld by citing a penological interest. One exception involved Nevada's mandatory testing policy, which was struck down based on lack of evidence of a legitimate interest.[24]

County Prison Response–Policy Changes

The county continues to modify its policy. It is now entitled "the infectious disease policy" rather than a specific policy for HIV/AIDS with the inclusion of guidelines about hepatitis and tuberculosis. The policy has also been modified to meet with legislative changes which require written informed consent prior to HIV testing.

Housing has also been revised to accommodate overcrowding:

> Once it is ascertained that an inmate is in a high risk category, the nursing staff is to be notified to obtain a blood sample. An

assessment of the inmate will be done by officers, counselors, or management with several questions in mind. Is the inmate aggressive? Does he/she have a history of violence? What are the past and present charges? What is the demeanor of the inmate? If a preliminary assessment determines that the inmate shows *potential* for aggressive behavior, double-lock, single celled until the test results are known. Officers are to use precautions inclusive of gloves, handcuffs, and nightsticks.

If an inmate is assessed to be cooperative and is non-aggressive, normal classification procedures will be followed. Once classification is complete, the inmate will be placed in general population. (County Prison, 1992 p. 10)

and:

Permanent housing shall be made on a case by case basis with several factors taken into consideration. These shall include: the medical and safety needs of the seropositive inmate, the security needs of the institution and housing availability. (p. 10)

Escorting inmates within the prison compound now resembles the procedure for general inmate population. Yet, an exception is listed for the disruptive HIV-positive inmate:

Inmates who show a poor attitude, poor behavior, or are assessed potentially aggressive will be transported by two officers. Precautionary measures will include gloves, handcuffs, and nightsticks. Modifications of these procedures may be made upon the improvement of the inmate's overall attitude and behavior. (County Prison, 1992, p. 10)

HIV-positive inmates are integrated into activities when their housing is general population although restrictions still apply to trustee status and work release. An appeal process has been incorporated into the policy for any HIV-positive inmate to protest a procedure. Most of these changes, though, were merely the writing down of what was being done daily.

Throughout the policy continuum, the correctional staff has remained the advantaged population. Policy changes, for the most part, evolved from complaints of workload. This was coupled with the administration's overcrowded conditions and the constant pressure to keep the budget under control. As stated with Schneider and Ingram (1993), the advantaged group remains powerful and their concerns are readily addressed in the arena of AIDS policy. Although authority tools of force could have been used (such as a suspension for refusal to follow procedure), incentive tools involving training and overtime pay aided in ensuring compliance.

The contenders were initially met with strong opposition, but due to the changing viewpoint of the staff, many were able to move their social construction into the advantaged group. The new contenders that emerged were those who opposed the current direction of the AIDS policy. This group was scattered and consisted of a few correctional officers, one or two supervisors, and a few members of management. Also, the ACLU became a contender representing the complaints of a former inmate. The prison administrators were very defensive of what they termed an innovative policy and were relieved when it was determined that the complaints were unfounded.

The dependents' viewpoint has also evolved. The inmate population still remains reliant on the advantaged officers to voice their concerns and to watch out for their needs. Yet, because HIV infection has spread among IV drug users, the general population has been much more sympathetic and accepting of seropositive inmates in the cell blocks. Many of the former deviant HIV-positive inmates now occupy the dependent category. They have proven to be no physical threat and have readily agreed to go along with the policy directives. Almost all the HIV-positive inmates have been quite concerned about infecting others and have taken extreme measures to prevent even casual contact with cellmates. Their cooperation and consideration has earned many of them a positive construction— which has allowed a move from the deviant category to the dependent group. They now can be viewed as "inmates with an illness." This signifies a monumental step forward.

Unfortunately, the deviant targets remain. Infected gay inmates are required to keep their sexual preference to themselves or have been forced to advance a different status such as IV drug user in order to gain acceptance. Today most officers and inmates remain homophobic and classify homosexual activity within the institution differently than the same choice outside the facility. Even gay inmates who are not infected carefully guard their personal lifestyle to avoid harassment and threats from others. The HIV-positive gay inmate is still blamed for his infection and little sympathy is evoked for pain and suffering.

The prostitute has also been accused for causing her infection. Despite evidence that risk is linked to IV drug use or lack of condom use in personal relationships, prostitutes have been presented as "vessels of transmission" (Hogan, 1994). The courts have been extremely harsh in sentencing HIV-positive prostitutes as well. Many times, the length of time has been equivalent to life imprisonment.

Finally, HIV-positive inmates incarcerated for the first time who are unknown to the staff or those who complain about the protocol remain burdened with restrictive measures. As for all HIV-infected inmates, any sign of a poor attitude or misbehavior can result in a quick change of status—back to the deviant category. Schneider and Ingram's model points out that punishment is deemed most appropriate for deviant constructions. Seropositive inmates with this negative construction are still viewed as less deserving of benefits and policy consideration.

Throughout the three periods of policy development, the four classifications provided by the Schneider and Ingram model have been apparent. The advantaged staff have been able to use their positive construction and their power to alter the course of AIDS correctional policy for their own benefit. This has been supported by administrators who have answered their concerns with funds for protective gear, testing, and identification of those infected. When this became a burden to the advantaged population, policy was again altered to meet their new demands.

Those who have been represented by the contender category have changed over time. Initially, the medical staff and a few prison personnel contested the harsh policies. Slowly they were able to transform their position by gaining increased staff support and backing from outside agencies. This allowed a shift from an adversarial position to a positively constructed image within the advantaged group. The emergence of a new contender group which opposed the incremental changes now clashed with the advantaged group. They were viewed negatively by the staff and dependents, but had enough influence to slow down or stall policy changes.

The general prison population has occupied the dependent category in AIDS policy but has been expanded to include many of the HIV-positive inmates. Although still undersubscribed in receiving benefits, burdens are enforced to protect them from harm (Schneider & Ingram; 1993).

Finally, the deviant classification remains for those infected who are viewed as misfits in the prison as well as society. Negatively constructed and powerless to change their status at this time, they continue to be the target for restrictive measures.

CONCLUSION

It is hard to adjust to being a deviant among an already deviant society. A certain amount of mistreatment is expected by most people incarcerated, but it is especially hard to adapt when both the officers and other inmates label someone as aberrant. Anyone facing HIV/AIDS is traumatized and fearful. The reality of how tentative life can be is immediately pushed to the forefront with an urgency to accomplish goals that were dreamed of over a long period of time. This in itself requires inner strength, and outer support from others. Imagine the difficulty of facing this disease behind bars. Those infected have no control over their lives, their goals, or their medical choices. They are deprived of paramour and family support and are left to deal with this disease in a hostile environment. Their fate is placed in the hands of officers, counselors, and the courts, who will determine how deserving they are of freedom in order to die with dignity.

Despite the evolution of AIDS policy in many institutions, the special needs and concerns of the HIV-positive inmate are displaced for greater institutional goals. Fear still dominates policy and the thought of allowing an inmate to have a voice is considered ludicrous. Yet, an exception must be made for those with terminal illnesses who do not present a danger to the staff, other inmates, or society.

The first step can be taken by allowing HIV-positive inmates active participation in AIDS policy formation and revision. Sec-

FIGURE 1. Variations in How Policy Treats Target Populations: Allocation of Benefits and Burdens

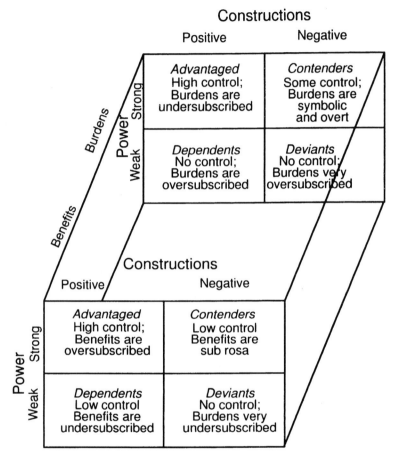

Note: Benefits are shown on the front part of the box to each type of target; burdens are shown at the back of the box.
Reprinted with Permission from *American Political Science Review.*

ondly, choices in medical treatment should be encouraged, including the allowance of participation in clinical trials of experimental drugs. Finally, efforts should be made to include HIV-positive inmates themselves in training and education programs—especially those directed at other inmates.

AIDS policy at the county prison remains the same with very few revisions expected. Other concerns have become more pressing and the needs of the seropositive inmates have faded into the background. The county prison's current policy, though, presents a much more open and humanistic approach than many correctional facilities. It must be demanded that harsh treatment out of ignorance and fear about the disease be eliminated through effective education and training for both the officers and the inmates and that administrators take a strong proactive stance in advancing humane procedures.

This essay was written to draw attention to the past and present treatment of HIV-positive inmates and to provide a voice which speaks with urgency–imploring that a more compassionate approach to AIDS correctional policy be instituted. Inclusion in the construction of prison-based AIDS policy will not only provide empowerment to the HIV-positive inmates but will encourage cooperative efforts to overcome fear and intolerance within the prison setting.

NOTES

1. Donovan (1994) states that it appears that only pharmaceutical companies fit the contender category. I would expand this to include those groups which are negatively constructed but have strong political power to advance their agendas such as Lambda Legal Defense (see Aiken & Musheno, 1994).

2. Donovan (1994) provides an excellent example of contender groups receiving sub-rosa policy benefits. The Ryan White Care Act of 1990 placed emphasis on providing aid to women and children while masking the receipt of these same benefits to the gay population.

3. Hemophiliacs are gaining power as a result of organizing nationally and are becoming politically active in AIDS policy.

4. Primarily advocates within the institution consisted of medical staff and inmate counselors.

5. The term general population is not being applied to identify a specific housing classification. Rather, it implies the inmates who are not infected with HIV.

6. These cases only represent a few of the lawsuits filed on behalf on the non-infected inmate population. For example, in Feigley v. Fulcomer, 720 F. Supp. 475, 481 (M.D. PA 1989), noninfected prisoners sued for inmate testing, whether voluntarily requested or mandatory. At the time, PA Department of Corrections provided no testing. In Glick v. Henderson, 855 F2d. 536 (8th Circ. 1988), the inmates wanted all prison personnel included in the mass screening of inmates. In

Jarrett v. Faulkner, 662 F. Supp 928 (S.D. Ind, 1987), noninfected prisoners wanted all inmates to be tested and HIV-positive inmates segregated from general population.

7. The window period refers to the period of time between becoming infected and the development of antibodies which are detected by the blood test. The average time of antibody formation is stated to be 6 to 12 weeks. Recommendations called for re-testing at 6 weeks, 3 months, 6 months, and 1 year after the initial screen (CDC, 1985).

8. AZT was approved for use on March 19, 1987, and introduced by Burroughs-Welcome on March 24, 1987. At this time, AZT was quite expensive. The expense was justified for ongoing research, but public pressure resulted in a price reduction on December 15, 1987, and again in 1989 (Burroughs-Welcome Company, 1995).

9. Seropositivity refers to having the presence of HIV antibodies.

10. The four states that used mass screening were Nevada, Colorado, Iowa, and Missouri.

11. Media reports from Florida stated that several individuals had become infected from "HIV-bearing" mosquitoes. Despite being disproved, the thought of the "unknown" prevailed, which heightened staff fear and anxiety (MMWR, 1986, p. 23). Also of concern were body fluids such as tears or spitting and possible transmission within food. (For a more complete explanation discounting these alternate modes of transmission, see Lifson, 1988; CDC, 1985; MMWR, 1985.)

12. Extra-institutional staff was not required to sign any documents which would ensure confidentiality of the inmates HIV status.

13. Blumberg (1989) cites two studies substantiating that homosexual activity exists in prison. Estimates range from 30% participation (Nacci & Kane, 1983, p. 35) to over 65% (Wooden & Parker, 1982, pp. 50-52). Both studies looked at male inmates only.

14. Initial instructions were to soak the handcuffs in bleach. All prison handcuffs had been dipped in copper to distinguish them from other transporting agencies cuffs. It was quickly realized the bleach removed the copper and corroded the cuffs. This resulted in a change in policy to wiping the handcuffs off with alcohol.

15. Hammett (1989) reports that the mean average for male IV drug use was 71% while 45% was attributed to homosexuality. For females, 95% of those infected were associated with IV drug use (p. 11).

16. In 1988, the highest concentrations of HIV-positive inmates were found in California, New York, New Jersey, and Pennsylvania.

17. The Centers for Disease Control conducted a study in Nevada which generated the rate of exposure as .17 percent per year (Hammett, 1989, p. 17).

18. Two claims had been made of occupational exposure. A correctional officer in Maricopa County (Phoenix), Arizona, reported a spitting incident. When investigated, it was found that the seropositivity was not job related. Another claim was made in Philadelphia, PA, but the officer left the employ of the facility and never followed up by filing a claim (Hammett, 1989, p. 8).

19. By 1990, the treatment with AZT per year averaged around $5,000. As of 1994, the average treatment based on five doses of 100 mg of AZT per day costs $2621 per year. Six doses per day costs $3,154 per year (Bartlett, 1994, p. 140).

20. At this time, HIV positivity was categorized as asymptomatic (HIV infected but no clinical symptoms or intermittent symptoms), ARC (AIDS-Related Complex where symptoms were recurring), and end stage AIDS (recurring symptoms with the development of opportunistic infections).

21. The concern of overcrowding was directly related to the policy goal of maintaining security. Most institutions were not adequately staffed to match the continuing increase in the inmate population.

22. Previous prison policy stated that isolation cells must be visually inspected every 15 minutes. The officer was then required to document his/her observations.

23. This was especially true with the women. Whenever an HIV-positive female was identified, the other inmates were empathetic and nurturing.

24. Walker v. Sumner, 917 F.2d 382 (9th Cir. 1990).

REFERENCES

Aiken, J., & Musheno, M. (1994). Why have-nots win in the HIV litigation arena: Socio-legal dynamics of extreme cases. *Law and Policy, 16*(3), 235-247.

Bartlett, J. (1994). *Medical management of HIV infection.* Glenview, IL: Physician and Scientist Publishing, Inc.

Bayer, R. (1989). *Private acts, social consequences: AIDS and the politics of public health.* New York: Free Press.

Belbot, B., & del Carmen, R. (1991). AIDS in prison: Legal issues. *Crime and Delinquency, 37*(1), 135-153.

Blumberg, M. (1989). Issues and controversies with respect to the management of AIDS in corrections. *The Prison Journal, 69*(1), 1-13.

Blumberg, M., & Langston, D. (1991). Mandatory HIV testing in criminal justice settings. *Crime and Delinquency, 37*(1), 5-18.

Burris, S. (1992). Prisons, law and public health: The case for a coordinated response to epidemic disease behind bars. *University of Miami Law Review, 47*(2), 291-335.

Burroughs-Welcome Company (February 27, 1995). Phone conversation with Drug Information Department.

Carroll, L. (1992). AIDS and human rights in the prison: A comment on the ethics of screening and segregation. In C. Hartjen & E. Rhine (Eds.), *Correctional theory and practice* (pp. 162-177). Chicago, IL: Nelson-Hall, Inc.

Centers for Disease Control. (1985). Recommendation for preventing transmission of infection with human t-lymphotropic virus type III/lymphadenopathy-associated virus in the workplace-summary. *Department of Health and Human Services,* November 15, pp. 681-686, 691-695.

Christensen, K. (1990). Prison issues and HIV: Introduction. In M. Banzhaf et al. (Eds.), *Women, AIDS, and activism* (pp. 139-142). Boston, MA: South End Press.

Cohen, J., Alexander P., & Wofsy, C. (1988). Prostitutes and AIDS: Public policy. issues. *AIDS and Public Policy Journal, 3*(2), 16-22.

County Prison. (1992). *Infectious disease policy.*

County Prison. (1990). *Policy on the management of HIV infection.*

County Prison. (1988). *Policy on the management of HIV infection.*

County Prison. (1987). *Policy on the management of HIV infection.*

Darrow, W. (1990). Prostitution, drugs, and HIV in the U.S. In M. Plant (Ed.), *AIDS, drugs, and prostitution* (pp. 18-40). New York: Tavistock/Routledge.

Donovan, M. (1994). Social constructions of people with AIDS: Target populations and the United States policy, 1981-1990, *Policy Studies Review, 13*, 3-29.

Dubler, N., & Sidel, V. (1991). AIDS and the prison system. In D. Nelkin, D. Willis, & S. Parris (Eds.), *A disease of society: Cultural and institutional responses to AIDS* (pp. 71-83). Cambridge, MA.: Cambridge University Press.

Gregware, P. (1994). Courts, criminal process, and AIDS: The institutionalization of culture in legal decision making. *Law and Policy, 16*(3), 342-362.

Hammett, T., Harrold L., Gross, M., & Epstein, J. (1994). *1992 Update: HIV/ AIDS in correctional facilities, issues and options.* Washington, DC: U.S. Government Printing Office.

Hammett, T., & Moini, S. (1990). *Update on AIDS in prisons and jails.* Washington, DC: U.S. Government Printing Office.

Hammett, T. (1989). *1988 Update: AIDS in correctional facilities.* Washington, DC: U.S. Government Printing Office.

Hammett, T. (1988). *AIDS in correctional facilities, issues and options* (3rd ed.). Washington, DC: U.S. Government Printing Office.

Hammett, T. (1986a). *AIDS in prisons and jails, issues and options.* Washington, DC: U.S. Government Printing Office.

Hammett, T. (1986b). *AIDS in correctional facilities, issues and options.* Washington, DC: U.S. Government Printing Office.

Hogan, N. (1994). HIV education for inmates: Uncovering strategies for program selection. *The Prison Journal, 74*(2), 220-243.

Ingram, H., & Schneider, A. (1991a). The choice of target populations. *Administration and Society, 23*(3), 333-356.

Ingram, H., & Schneider, A. (1991b). Improving implementation through framing smarter statutes. *Journal of Public Policy, 10*(1), 67-88.

JAMA Board of Trustees. (1987). Prevention and control of acquired immunodeficiency syndrome. *Journal of the American Medical Association, 258*, 2097-2103.

Jones, A., & Bishop, P. (1990). Policy making by the lower federal courts and the bureaucracy: The genesis of a national AIDS policy. *The Social Science Journal, 27*(3), 273-288.

Jurik, N., & Musheno, M. (1986). The internal crisis of corrections: Professionalization and the work environment. *Justice Quarterly, 32*, 457-480.

Leonard, Z., & Thistlethwaite, P. (1990). Prostitution and HIV infection. In M. Banzhof et al. (Eds.), *Women, AIDS, and activism* (pp. 177-185). Boston, MA: South End Press.

Lifson, A. (1988). Do alternate modes for transmission of human immunodeficiency virus exist? *Journal of the American Medical Association, 259*(9), 1353-1356.

Martin, R., & Zimmerman, S. (1990). Adopting precautions against HIV infection among male prisoners: A behavioral and policy analysis. *Criminal Justice Policy and Review, 4*(4), 330-348.

MMWR. (1987). *Recommendations for prevention of HIV transmission in health-care settings.*[Supplement]. DHHS, Washington, DC: U.S. Government Printing Office. August 21, 36: 2-18.

MMWR. (1986). Acquired immunodeficiency syndrome (AIDS) in western Palm Beach County, Florida. *Reports on AIDS, June 1986-May 1987.* DHHS, Washington, DC: U.S. Government Printing Office. October 3, 35: 609-612.

MMWR. (1985). Recommendations for preventing possible transmission Of Human T-Lymphotropic Virus Type III/Lymphadenopathy-Associated Virus from tears. *Reports of AIDS Published in the Morbidity and Mortality Weekly Report, June 1981 through May 1986.* DHHS, Washington, DC: U.S. Government Printing Office. August, 30, 34: 533-534.

Nacci, P., & Kane, T. (1983). The incidence of sex and sexual aggression in federal prisons. *Federal Probation, 47*, 31-36.

Olivero, J. (1989). Intravenous drug use and AIDS: A review and analysis of evolving correctional policy. *Criminal Justice Policy and Review, 3*(4), 360-375.

Olivero, J., & Roberts, J. (1989). The management of AIDS within correctional facilities: A view from the federal Courts. *The Prison Journal, 69*(2), 9-20.

Porter, V. (1988). Minorities and HIV infection. *New England Journal of Public Policy* [Special Issue on AIDS], 371-379.

Ross, J. (1988). Ethics and the language of AIDS. In C. Pierce & D. Vandeveer (Eds.), *AIDS ethics and public policy* (pp. 39-48). Belmont, CA: Wadsworth Publishing.

Schneider, A., & Ingram, H. (1994). Social construction and policy design: Implications for public administration. In J. Perry (Ed.), *Research in public administration,* Vol. 3 (pp. 137-173). Greenwich, CT: JAI Press.

Schneider, A., & Ingram, H. (1993). Social construction of target populations: Implications for politics and policy. *American Political Science Review, 87*(2), 334-347.

Schneider, A., & Ingram, H. (1990a). Behavioral assumptions of policy tools. *Journal of Politics, 52*(2), 510-529.

Schneider, A., & Ingram, H. (1990b). Policy design: Elements, premises, and strategies. In S. Nagel (Ed.), *Policy theory and policy evaluation* (pp. 77-101). New York: Greenwood Press.

Takas, M., & Hammett, T. (1989). Legal issues affecting offenders and staff. *AIDS Bulletin.* Washington, DC: U.S. Government Printing Office.

Turner, C., Miller, H., & Moses, L. (1989). *AIDS: Sexual behavior and intravenous drug use.* Washington, DC: National Academy Press.

Vlahov, D. (1990). HIV-1 infection in the correctional setting. *Criminal Justice Policy and Review, 4*(4), 306-318.

World Health Communications. (1988). *Rationale for antiviral therapy of HIV disease: An overview.* [brochure]. New York: World Health Communications, December.

Wooden, D., & Parker, J. (1982). *Men behind bars: Sexual exploitation in prison.* New York: Plenum Press.

COURT CASES

Feigley v. Fulcomer, 720 F. Supp. 475. 481 (M.D. PA 1989).
Glick v. Henderson, 855 F2d 536 (8th Circ. 1988).
Jarrett v. Faulkner, 622 F. Supp. 928 (S.D. Ind 1987).
Walker v. Sumner, 917 F.2d 382 (9th Cir. 1990).

The Problem
with Making AIDS Comfortable:
Federal Policy Making
and the Rhetoric of Innocence

Mark C. Donovan, PhD (cand.)

University of Washington

SUMMARY. This essay presents a narrative of U.S. AIDS policy which highlights the ways that people with AIDS (PWAs) have been categorized throughout the epidemic. I argue that PWAs have been broadly categorized as either "innocent" or "guilty" in the public discourse about AIDS, and that these distinctions have greatly influenced the way that policies are designed and justified. An examination of the Ryan White CARE Act of 1990 shows that policy rationales of lawmakers overwhelmingly relied on rhetoric which focused on the most sympathetic PWAs: "innocent" women and children. While this rhetorical strategy helped gain passage of the law, it effectively shut out the concerns of the majority of PWAs who

Mark C. Donovan is a doctoral candidate in the Department of Political Science at the University of Washington. His dissertation analyzes the connection between the design of health policies and policy rationales used by lawmakers to justify them.

The author would like to thank Michael Hallett, Dia Lautenschlager, and Peter May for their helpful comments on earlier versions of this manuscript.

Correspondence may be addressed: Department of Political Science, Box 353530, University of Washington, Seattle, WA 98195.

[Haworth co-indexing entry note]: "The Problem with Making AIDS Comfortable: Federal Policy Making and the Rhetoric of Innocence." Donovan, Mark C. Co-published simultaneously in *Journal of Homosexuality* (The Haworth Press, Inc.) Vol. 32, No. 3/4, 1997, pp. 115-144; and: *Activism and Marginalization in the AIDS Crisis* (ed: Michael A. Hallett) The Haworth Press, Inc., 1997, pp. 115-144; and: *Activism and Marginalization in the AIDS Crisis* (ed: Michael A. Hallett) Harrington Park Press, an imprint of The Haworth Press, Inc., 1997, pp. 115-144. Single or multiple copies of this article are available for a fee from The Haworth Document Delivery Service [1-800-342-9678, 9:00 a.m. - 5:00 p.m. (EST). E-mail address: get info@haworth.com].

115

fell into less sympathetic categories and resulted in policy decisions which often work against the stated goals of lawmakers. *[Article copies available for a fee from The Haworth Document Delivery Service: 1-800-342-9678. E-mail address: getinfo@haworth.com]*

There is ample evidence that popular discourse about AIDS in the United States has changed dramatically over its brief and devastating history. Initially AIDS was seen as an epidemic plague stoppable by emergency measures, and as is often the case during plagues, sickness was seen as a sign of guilt and deviance. A variety of factors forced amendments to the initial perceptions of HIV/ AIDS and of people with AIDS, and over time the discourse came to be dominated by the message that "everyone is at risk." But even as well-meaning public service messages proclaim that "AIDS does not discriminate," debate over AIDS policy continues to be animated, often subtly, sometimes quite explicitly, by claims about the deservedness and culpability of people with AIDS. The public struggle over political language, in its crudest form a competition between images of "guilty HIV carriers" and "innocent victims of AIDS," has important real world effects that must be investigated and considered if one hopes to understand and influence the politics and policy of HIV/AIDS.

This essay explores the different ways in which people with AIDS (PWAs) have been publicly grouped and characterized and argues that these socially constructed stereotypes have set the contours of AIDS policy in the United States. My central point is that the continued failure of U.S. AIDS policy to address the needs of citizens who are gay men or injection drug users is, in part, the ironic result of efforts to generate support for PWAs by promoting a vision of the epidemic which emphasized sympathetic sufferers. This effort to make AIDS a publicly comfortable issue results in a policy debate where important stakeholders are silenced and policies are too often governed by symbols rather than by logic or deliberation.

I begin this essay by discussing key sources of the social construction of people with AIDS in order to show that the initial constructions of PWAs presented them as being deviant and guilty. I pay particular attention to how these early—and, I would argue, still dominant—stereotypes have been supplemented by kinder and gentler images of PWAs. In the second section I briefly outline a promising framework for analyzing the relationship between groups targeted by public policies and the design of those policies. In the third section I draw upon my earlier account and use this framework to examine the Ryan White Comprehensive AIDS Resource Emergency (C.A.R.E.) Act of 1990, the first piece of federal legislation to provide for the care and treatment of people with AIDS. Here I examine both the design of the legislation as well as the debate surrounding its passage, and analyze the association between the social construction of different PWA target populations and the policy provisions aimed at them. My central argument throughout is that while the passage of the Ryan White Act was made possible by promoting images of "deserving victims of AIDS," this rhetorical strategy also served to reinforce the negative constructions of the majority of PWAs. I conclude by discussing the costs of such a strategy.

PLACING BLAME: CONSTRUCTING PEOPLE WITH AIDS

While the point can be made with far more nuance (e.g., Patton 1990; Crimp, 1988), the dominant image of people with AIDS has been that of the deviant gay male or injection drug user whose predicament is deserved. This construction of people with AIDS is very much bound up with the construction of AIDS itself. Noting that AIDS is a socially constructed phenomena does not deny the reality that HIV is an infectious virus which most often results in the death of those it infects. Rather, my point is to focus on how our representations of this condition are invested with certain qualities and to investigate the effect of these representations on policy making. While the social construction of images of AIDS and PWAs has been and continues to be a complex and dynamic process, three aspects of this process stand out. First, the definition and categorization of HIV/AIDS by medical professionals determined, in important ways, how target populations would be identified. Second, the discovery of AIDS set in motion historically familiar responses to disease and epidemics which centered on placing blame. Third, latent cultural stereotypes of the groups to which many PWAs can be said to belong profoundly influenced the shape of policies targeted at these groups. These three aspects of the construction of PWAs go a long way toward explaining the deviance and guilt attached to the most prevalent images of people with AIDS.

Defining AIDS

The decisions and responses of professionals involved in AIDS policy making played a significant role in the social construction of target populations. First, the determination of the official definition of AIDS by public health officials prompted a particular set of public responses to the epidemic. "AIDS" is not a disease, but rather is a syndrome: an umbrella designation for a condition marked by an immune system destroyed by HIV and invaded by any of a number of opportunistic infections. To "have AIDS" means that a person has tested HIV-positive and suffers from an infection on the list of "official" AIDS infections. The definition of AIDS underwent significant revisions in 1985, 1987, and 1993. This definition has substantive importance because it determines who qualifies for government benefits and serves to shape who, quite literally, becomes an AIDS statistic. These statistics, in turn, shape how elites and the public conceive of people with AIDS, and serve to both include and exclude different groups from policy makers' consideration. The most notable example is the failure of official AIDS definitions to include the gynecological manifestations of the syndrome, thus excluding many women from the definition, limiting their access to services, and misstating the character of the epidemic (Corea, 1992). The de facto exclusion of women from the definition of AIDS further bolstered the early stereotypes of PWAs as gay men and IDUs, reinforcing skewed perceptions of the epidemic.

Even if the AIDS definition had been more inclusive from the beginning, the classification of AIDS as a sexually transmitted disease contributed in important ways to the dominant constructions of PWAs. Though HIV can be contracted in a variety of nonsexual ways, AIDS has been classified as a sexually transmitted disease rather than as a viral disease. Instead of labeling AIDS a viral disease such as hepatitis B, which is transmittable in most of the same ways as HIV, AIDS has been categorized as a sexually transmitted disease (STD) much like syphilis or gonorrhea (Fernando, 1993, pp. 16-38; Gilman, 1988, p. 247). This is significant because, as Allan Brandt notes in his social history of venereal disease in America, "Medical and social values continue to define venereal disease as a uniquely sinful disease, indeed, to transform the disease into an indication of moral decay" (Brandt, 1985, p. 186). Thus the medical definition of AIDS as an STD practically insured that issues such as prevention and treatment would involve a policy debate centering on moral as well as medical judgments.

Scripts of Disease and Epidemics

The medical response to AIDS is intertwined with familiar historical scripts of epidemic and disease which have centered on allocating blame; at a very basic level the initial public response to the AIDS epidemic was a decidedly traditional one. The response followed an archetypal pattern beginning with the slow revelation of the existence of the epidemic, progressing to a stage where infection was equated with moral failing, and ultimately eliciting policy initiatives intended to restore the pre-epidemic order (Rosenberg, 1989).[1] This patterned response was undoubtedly accelerated by modern communications technology. One pair of scholars dubbed this mass-mediated epidemic the first "living-room epidemic" where the revelation of a spreading contagion came not with a firsthand exposure to the epidemic's effects but through television images of AIDS sufferers (Cook & Colby, 1992).

As with those infected during past epidemics, PWAs came to be seen as belonging to one of two groups. Most were regarded as blameworthy "carriers of AIDS," whereas a much smaller number came to be viewed as the "innocent victims of AIDS." As Dorothy Nelkin and Sander Gilman note, the relationship between devastating disease and the compulsion to assign blame for the devastation is age-old. They write that, "Clinical categories . . . are frequently associated with specific groups—sometimes identified by race, sometimes by nationality or social class. In each case, blame for disease turns into a crusade against those who are feared or who, by being different, are viewed as a threat to the established social order" (Nelkin & Gilman, 1991, p. 45).

The policy ramifications of such innocent/guilty labels can be seen in the federal response to syphilis at the beginning of this century. Syphilitic male soldiers were framed as the patriotic victims of disease-carrying prostitutes who, through their ostensibly willful infection of the fighting force, were implicitly collaborating with the enemy (Fee, 1988). Placing infected individuals into such moral categories has a clear influence on the policies aimed not just at infected individuals but also at the groups to which these infected persons are said to belong. Prostitutes during World War I became seen as more than mere collaborators with the enemy, they were effectively identified as the enemy. Labeled "venereal carriers," over 30,000 prostitutes were detained by Congressional order in government sponsored institutions during World War I (Brandt, 1988). This policy response was echoed by elected officials confronting the AIDS epidemic when suggestions of the quarantining and mass firings of gays were reportedly discussed within the Reagan Administration (Altman, 1986, p. 64).

Marginalizing the Marginalized

While the historical scripts for responding to epidemics and the classification of AIDS as a sexually transmitted disease provided an almost unconsciously accepted set of social constructions of PWAs, the force of cultural stereotypes of the groups associated with HIV/AIDS—most notably the popular images of gay men and injection drug users—had a profound influence on the formation of policies to combat the epidemic. Public health officials initially dubbed what would come to be known as AIDS a "gay cancer," and then later "Gay Related Immune Disorder" (G.R.I.D.): choices which forged an early and lasting link between homosexuality and infection. As the public health establishment distanced itself from emphasizing "risk group" and focused instead on "risk behaviors," people with AIDS have instead been categorized according to the probable context of HIV transmission—"homosexual sex," "illegal drug use," "blood transfusion," and so forth. While these designations may make sense for the purpose of collecting epidemiological data and targeting prevention efforts, they also serve to provide important cues to elites and the public about how to regard particular groups of PWAs.

The appearance of HIV/AIDS in already marginalized groups reinforced the tendency to identify sickness with moral failing and seemed to insure that the dominant image of PWAs would be that of the guilty deviant. The stigma of disease and the stigma of homosexuality, in particular, were often conflated. As Allan Brandt notes, "In this context, homosexuality–not a virus–*causes* AIDS. Therefore homosexuality itself is feared as if it were a communicable, lethal disease" (Brandt, 1991, p. 107, emphasis in original). That not all PWAs were gay only highlighted the culpability of those who were. A 1983 *New York Times Magazine* article noted, for example, that "The groups most recently found to be at risk for AIDS present a particularly poignant problem," hemophiliacs, transfusion recipients, and babies were "innocent bystanders caught in the path of a new disease" (Brandt, 1988, p. 165). The "innocence" of these "bystanders" makes sense only in relation to a vision of guilty participants. The "poignant problem" was that of sorting the innocent minority from the guilty majority.

Sorting People with AIDS

In the mid-1980s concrete images of "innocents with AIDS" were presented to the American public and the rise of "innocents" as a pervasive construction of some people with AIDS became the most important supplement to the prevailing constructions of PWAs as sexual deviants or drug addicts. The conventional wisdom, expressed by journalist Randy Shilts (1987, p. 585), is "that there were two clear phases to the disease in the United States: there was AIDS before Rock Hudson and AIDS after." This common observation has been confirmed by Rogers, Dearing, and Chang (1991), who found that it was Hudson's 1985 disclosure that he was suffering from AIDS–rather than a change in the character of the epidemic or the introduction of new information about AIDS–that led to a permanent increase in media attention to the disease and thus increased the exposure of the public to news of the epidemic. Kinsella (1989) similarly argues that media coverage of AIDS has been tied to the extent to which the threat to "mainstream" Americans was perceived to be increasing, rather than to empirical indicators such as the epidemic's death toll.

Though Hudson's announcement is commonly viewed as a milestone, the media coverage of Ryan White's exclusion from school in Kokomo, Indiana, and his battle to return to the classroom cannot be ignored. The two media events occurred nearly simultaneously: the official Hudson announcement came on July 23, 1985, following weeks of speculation; the first Ryan White story appeared on network television on July 31 followed by several reports from all three networks in the next month (Nagle, 1989). The increased media attention to AIDS which immediately followed this joint event consisted of more than just stories about the two figures—in fact news stories about Rock Hudson and Ryan White accounted together for less than half of the increase in news stories about AIDS. The event put AIDS on the media agenda and "changed the meaning of the issue of AIDS for media newspeople, and ultimately for the American people" (Rogers, Dearing, & Chang, 1991, p. 13).

The case of Hudson is particularly instructive because one would not necessarily imagine that, as a gay man, his announcement would force a reconsideration of PWAs. Paula Treichler has observed, though, that many in the media and public could not reconcile Hudson's masculine screen persona with news of his homosexuality. She suggests that news stories attempted to "normalize" Hudson and cites as an example a *USA Today* article on the event in which a man is quoted saying "I thought AIDS was a gay disease, but if Rock Hudson can get it, anyone can" (Treichler, 1988, pp. 205, 249-250). For many, it seems, it was easier to think of AIDS as no longer just a "gay disease" than it was to reconcile deep stereotypes about homosexuality.

The Ryan White story also challenged the prevailing construction of PWAs. White, a hemophiliac, appeared on television as a relatively healthy looking young teen, and through his activism and many media appearances became the personification of the message that "anyone can get AIDS." But the incongruity of a child with AIDS did not instantly dispel fears of AIDS and the accompanying stereotypes of PWAs. In a typographical error which seems to confirm this confusion, one newspaper ran a photo of White in 1986 noting that he was a "homophiliac" (Gilman, 1988, p. 268). Still, the image of a child with AIDS—and of this child being discriminated against because of AIDS—was a powerful one. Like the troubling images of a dying Rock Hudson, Ryan White's story created dissonance within the public discourse about AIDS.[2]

The challenge to the dominant image of PWAs was coupled with a renewed fear of AIDS. A study of newspaper coverage of the epidemic found that "articles from 1985 [the time of the Hudson/ White stories] and 1986 reawakened fear of contagion and death. But those fears were now democratized, suggesting that AIDS's impact impinged on the daily lives of everyone–women, babies, students, workers, people dating, etc." (Albert, 1989, p. 49). The incongruities between non-gay, non-injection drug using PWAs and prevailing stereotypes did not, however, lead to a reassessment of the negative construction of gays and IDUs with AIDS, but instead led to the creation of new, identifiable groups of PWAs such as "women with AIDS" and "children with AIDS."

This shift in the public categorization of PWAs is crucial to the history of AIDS policy making, because for the first time these new categories of people with AIDS provided lawmakers and public advocates with sympathetic symbols of the AIDS crisis. As I argue below, the passage of the Ryan White Act was facilitated in many important ways by the creation of new, ostensibly more deserving categories of people with AIDS. Prior to this shift lawmakers did not perceive the extension of benefits to PWAs as defensible in light of the prevailing negative image of AIDS sufferers. Nevertheless, it is important not to be misled by this "improvement" in the image of some PWAs, for as the fear of AIDS was "democratized" the policy response was not. Even as public discourse has come to stress the egalitarian threat of AIDS and to emphasize its "victims," public policies continue to selectively reinscribe judgments of guilt, a process we must understand if we hope to change it.

A FRAMEWORK FOR ANALYSIS

To this point I have suggested that throughout the AIDS epidemic people with AIDS have been publicly grouped and characterized in ways that have important implications for how they are regarded by the public, but I have only alluded to the connection between these public characterizations and policy making. The connection between pervasive stereotypes and public policy making is at the center of a recent framework for social construction analysis proposed by Anne Schneider and Helen Ingram (1993). They present a model of policy making which holds that both the justifications for and the substance of public policies can be broadly predicted by understanding the social construction and political power of the groups being targeted by a given policy. In this section I outline the Schneider and Ingram perspective, and in the next I use it to frame my analysis of the Ryan White Act.

Schneider and Ingram present a model in which identifiable groups of actors or target populations are imbued with culturally constructed positive or negative images which influence the types of policy benefits and burdens lawmakers are willing to aim at them. When reelection concerns drive policy making, public officials must be certain that their policy choices—including the selection of target populations to receive benefits and burdens—will maximize their electoral advantage (Schneider & Ingram, 1993, pp. 335-337). Therefore, public officials can be expected to make policies which treat groups in ways which conform to dominant societal stereotypes. For the most part this means that politicians attempt to bestow benefits on positively constructed groups and burdens on negatively constructed populations. But in addition to the social valence of a particular group, politicians must also be aware of the relative political power of various populations. Powerful, positively constructed populations—the "advantaged"—and powerless, negatively constructed populations—the "deviant"—represent congruent, political ideal types. Politicians can bolster their electoral advantage by conferring benefits on advantaged groups and dumping burdens on deviant ones. When the powerless are positively constructed or, more troublesome for the politician, when powerful groups are negatively constructed, policy decisions become less straightforward. Although policy makers must present a "believable causal logic connecting the various aspects of the policy design to desired outcomes," there are often multiple ways to frame an issue, allowing legislators to exploit strategies which maximize the benefits and minimize the burdens targeted at preferred groups (Schneider & Ingram, 1993, p. 336).

Schneider and Ingram's typology of target populations simplifies a complex reality by holding that four key types of target populations are defined by the intersections of social construction (dichotomized as positive or negative) and political power (dichotomized as high or low). This typology is presented in Table 1. Groups

TABLE 1. Schneider and Ingram's Typology of Target Populations*

	Positive Construction	Negative Construction
Politically Powerful	**Advantaged** Receive mainly benefits Rarely receive burdens High control of agenda	**Contenders** Benefits tend to be hidden Burdens often symbolic Some agenda control
Politically Powerless	**Dependents** Benefits often symbolic Also receive some burdens Some agenda control	**Deviants** Rarely receive benefits Receive mainly burdens No control of the agenda

*Adapted from Schneider and Ingram (1993)

having a relatively large degree of political power and predominantly positive image to society are more likely to receive benefits when targeted by public policies and, as a result of both direct political power and the symbolic leverage accompanying their popular image, have a relatively high degree of control over the shape of policies selecting them as targets. Groups having a relatively large degree of political power but a predominantly negative public image—"contenders"—have little control over the distribution of policy benefits, but retain some degree of control over the shape of policy burdens. In view of their negative public construction they are likely to be the subject of at least some symbolic burdens while any benefits conferred by a policy will generally be delivered sub rosa or justified by an attempt to generalize the benefit, arguing, for example, that it is "in the national interest."

The typology of target populations is completed by two additional categories of groups, each possessing little political power. "Dependent" groups are more likely to receive burdens than benefits, but given their prevailing positive construction these groups may be able to exert some leverage on the policy process in order to be targeted for some policy benefits. These benefits, though, are likely to be symbolic rather than substantive. Deviant groups are also likely to receive burdens rather than benefits, but lacking power and a positive construction, deviants are unlikely to be able to influence policy in ways beneficial to them. Under Schneider and Ingram's schema, people with AIDS fit into either the dependent or deviant cell. Women, children, hemophiliacs, and blood transfusion recipients are generally constructed as dependents, while gays and injection drug users (IDUs) are labeled deviant. It needs to be stressed that these are not hard and fast designations. The position of gays in the matrix of target populations has shifted over time as the gay community politically mobilized its members, which increased its political profile but did not eradicate the negative constructions of gay men with AIDS.

Schneider and Ingram's typology is useful because it gives researchers and activists a framework for systematically unpacking key influences on the policy making process. Furthermore, it helps to explain inequalities in the distribution of benefits and burdens to different groups and illustrates the important connections between political language and public policy. Such an analysis is especially useful in a case like AIDS where rhetoric is so charged and the stakes are so high. In the next section I use the Schneider and Ingram typology to guide the analysis of a landmark piece of AIDS legislation, the Ryan White Act, where the potent symbolism of "dependent" populations and the difficult position of "deviant" populations is clear.

THE RYAN WHITE C.A.R.E. ACT

The importance of taking into account the social constructions of target populations is bluntly illustrated by examining the Ryan White Comprehensive AIDS Resource Emergency Act.[3] Passed in 1990, the act was the first piece of comprehensive AIDS legislation designed to deliver treatment and care to people with AIDS. The way in which passage of the act was justified by lawmakers and the way the act distributed burdens and benefits to various groups of PWAs supports Schneider and Ingram's typology of target populations and, more importantly for my argument, illuminates the ways in which political constraints hamper the adoption of reasonable public policies.

The Bill

Passage of the law was made possible by events which helped to broaden the public conception of who is at risk for HIV infection. In their public statements lawmakers overwhelmingly relied on the rationale that the act would take care of the "innocent victims" of AIDS. I argue that the shift in public consciousness about PWAs that had its origins in the media attention surrounding Rock Hudson and Ryan White provided an opportunity for policy makers to construct AIDS policy which could deliver benefits to "deserving" target populations. Prior to this shift, lawmakers did not perceive the extension of care and treatment to PWAs as a defensible policy in light of the prevailing image of AIDS sufferers and their own focus on reelection.

At the time the Ryan White Act was considered, potential PWA target populations were arrayed along the continuums of political power and positive/negative construction in a manner illustrated in Figure 1. The percent of the total PWAs represented by each group in 1990 is noted in parentheses in the figure. There is, of course, some overlapping membership between some groups (for instance, gay men who inject drugs). This arrangement of target populations is based on a review of a wide range of published analysis and commentary on the epidemic.[4]

While the absolute position of groups is to some extent arbitrary, the relative position of each population is not. Injection drug users anchor the lower right hand corner of the space with an extremely negative image and no political power. The political mobilization of the gay community and an increasingly favorable (though still predominantly negative) public image is noted by the up and leftward movement of the gay community. Women and racial and ethnic minorities are located on the social construction continuum somewhere between drug users and children as their infection still conveys to many evidence of a moral failing. They are positioned relatively low on the power continuum because as a group their political mobilization has lagged behind the gay community and advocates for children. Children, hemophiliacs, and blood transfusion recipients are all positively constructed. Children, by virtue of the political mobilization of pediatric AIDS lobbying groups and

FIGURE 1. Distribution of PWA Target Populations, 1990
(Percentage of total AIDS cases by category in parentheses)

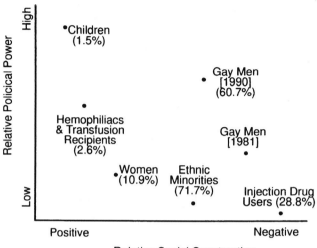

Sources: See note 3. AIDS case data from National Research Council,
1990, pp. 44, 51, 55. Percentages sum to over 100% as a result of overlapping group membership.

the prevailing sympathy for their plight, are positioned as the most politically powerful of these groups.

The House version of the Ryan White CARE Act (HR 4785) was sponsored by Henry Waxman (D-Calif.) and the Senate version (S 2240) was introduced by Edward Kennedy (D-Mass.). Both bills passed with overwhelming bipartisan support, though the subsequent failure of the Congress to fully fund the act suggests that much of this support was purely symbolic. The House bill cleared the chamber on June 13, 1990, with a vote of 408-14. The Senate version passed a month earlier on May 16, 95-4. The markup period in the House Subcommittee on Health and the Environment, chaired by Waxman, and the floor debate in both houses were spent considering a variety of restrictive amendments offered by Republican lawmakers. Amendments requiring states to develop partner notification programs and forbidding the use of grants to fund needle exchange programs were adopted in response to more restrictive amendments offered by Representative William Dannemeyer (R-Calif.) and Senator Jesse Helms (R-N.C.), respectively. The conference report was adopted by both houses on August 4, 1990. The final version of the bill authorized $875 million in fiscal 1991 and was signed into law by President Bush on August 18 (*Congressional Quarterly Almanac*, 1990).

As passed, the Ryan White Act provides emergency relief grants to cities with more than 2,000 reported cases of AIDS, HIV-care grants to states to provide health and support services to HIV-positive individuals, and funding for early intervention services for persons who have contracted or are at risk to contract HIV. The act specifies that fifteen percent of the HIV-care grants are to be set aside to provide services to infants, children, women, and families with AIDS, and up to ten percent of the grants are to be spent on special projects such as delivering services to hemophiliacs or Native Americans with AIDS. It is important to note that these set-asides are not congruent with the number of PWAs in these target populations. The final version of the law also contained provisions requiring states to develop programs to notify the sexual partners of persons testing HIV-positive, prohibited the use of federal funds to provide clean needles to injection drug users, and required states to adopt laws criminalizing the intentional transmission of HIV. Funds were authorized to pay for the mandatory testing of prisoners convicted of sex-related crimes, demonstration projects to improve treatment and services to infants and children with AIDS, a study of AIDS in rural areas, and grants to implement emergency-worker guidelines designed to reduce the risk of on-the-job HIV infection.

The Debate

The Senate floor debate on the Ryan White Act highlights the differentiation of PWA target populations which occurred on both sides of the aisle. Senator David Pryor (D-Ark.) seems to distinguish the deserving PWAs from those who might not be as deserving: "[PWAs] are not necessarily homosexuals and once again they are not from San Francisco or just New York. They are children whose only sin is to be born" (U.S. Congress, Senate, 1990a, p. S6193). The implication, of course, is that homosexuals are guilty of other sins. Despite the fact that the vast majority of the reported AIDS cases in 1990 were among gays and IDUs, Jesse Helms argued that the act should be focused on more deserving, dependent populations:

> My point is that this legislation should focus on the 2 percent [of PWAs] like Ryan White and like that young woman surgeon from Puerto Rico [who received a tainted blood transfusion]. It should focus on the women and children. (U.S. Congress, Senate, 1990a, p. S6197)

While the act as passed ultimately distributed the bulk of its funding to states to use for undifferentiated spending for the care and treatment of PWAs, it did contain a mix of provisions targeted at specific populations. Under the act, deviant PWAs are the subject of policy burdens. Prisoners convicted of sex-related crimes are required to undergo mandatory HIV testing (though no treatment or care funds were targeted at prisoners), IDUs are prohibited from being given clean needles, and the knowing *possible* transmission of HIV is a crime. Each of these coercive provisions is a watered-down version of much stricter sanctions: the original proposal for prisoner testing called for the mandatory testing of all prisoners regardless of crime, an amendment to ban even the distribution of bleach to IDUs in order to allow them to clean their needles and syringes was proposed, and the initial amendment to criminalize the possible transmission of HIV specifically targeted drug users and prostitutes regardless of their HIV status. This later amendment introduced by Senator Helms would have made it a crime to donate blood if an individual

> who, on or after January 1, 1977 is or has been a user of any intravenous drug . . . [or] has engaged in prostitution. . . . Transmission of the Human Immuno-deficiency Virus *does not have to occur* [emphasis added] for a person to have committed a violation of this section. (U.S. Congress, Senate, 1990b, p. S6294)

This amendment would have penalized individuals based solely on their affiliation with a deviant group rather than on their transmission of HIV as, under this language, an HIV-person could be convicted.

The amendment was introduced by Helms as the "Ryan White Amendment" and is an excellent example of a policy being crafted to seemingly provide a generalized benefit (a safe blood supply) while placing burdens on deviants. It was narrowly defeated (47-52), but what is most interesting is that the rationales offered by opponents of the amendment had little to do with the merits of the amendment as a public health measure. The reasoning most commonly asserted in opposition to the amendment was that it might incorrectly assign rehabilitated, "normalized" individuals to a deviant population. Senator Kennedy contended that the amendment would penalize people "who are now completely reformed," while Senator Carl Levin (D-Mich.) echoed this logic noting that an individual who "successfully underwent drug rehabilitation" could be labeled a criminal if the Helms amendment passed (U.S. Congress, Senate, 1990b, pp. S6301, S6304). As the Schneider and Ingram perspective suggests, there was no disagreement that deviants should be the target of sanctions, only disagreement as to how to properly identify members of those populations in order to maintain the boundaries separating the deserving from the undeserving. Under the act, small special project grants were established to improve drug treatment programs, but given the burdens placed on IDUs elsewhere in the act, these treatment grants are largely symbolic and serve to bolster the opinions expressed above that IDUs can and should be rehabilitated and reformed. The extension of symbolic grants, I would argue, reinforces the prevailing social construction of IDUs as deviants whose personal culpability now includes a failure to take advantage of government assistance.

Deviants were not the only set of target populations differentiated under the Ryan White Act; dependents found themselves designated the recipients of some symbolic and substantive policy benefits. Although nearly 90 percent of the AIDS cases reported through 1990 were among adult men, the Ryan White Act required that 15 percent of the Title II, HIV-care grants be set aside for women and children. This disproportionate funding was justified on the grounds that pediatric AIDS was more expensive than adult AIDS, and that these two populations represented some of the fastest growing segments of the AIDS epidemic. Yet this rationale willfully ignores the previous failures to provide funding for IDUs and inner-city blacks and Hispanics, who represent a huge, growing population with AIDS. The perceived deviance of IDUs explains their neglect by lawmakers, and the lack of political power possessed by inner-city PWAs accounts for the absence of set-asides for that population.

In contrast, advocates for children with AIDS are relatively well funded and well organized. Their concerns are presented to Congress by groups such as the Pediatric AIDS Foundation, the Pediatric AIDS Coalition, and the National Hemophilia Foundation. The clout and the positive construction of this dependent population is witnessed by the fact that of the 17 Congressional hearings on AIDS which took place in the three years leading up to the passage of the Ryan White Act, four (24%) focused exclusively on pediatric AIDS. None of the hearings focused similarly on gay men or IDUs and only two centered on the problems of AIDS in the inner city. Though ostensibly advocates for all children with AIDS, the children most often the subject of Congressional attention have been "the children with hemophilia or children who have received transfusions, not the children of heroin-injecting minority mothers" (National Research Council, 1993, p. 211). Apparently the innocent/guilty dichotomy also serves to sort children with AIDS.

The inordinate focus on "innocent" children with AIDS can be seen as reflecting a legislative strategy used by lawmakers intent on publicized public concern for children with AIDS. Public officials do not simply react to social constructions floating in the ether, but often seek to privilege certain constructions in order to achieve political and policy goals. Despite the women and children set-aside, the majority of the care and treatment funds authorized under the act would ultimately be translated into services delivered to gay men, who in 1990 comprised over half of the documented cases of AIDS. Unlike spending for AIDS research, which allocates funds to a positively constructed biomedical research establishment and, in the best case, produces results which are long-lasting and widely dispersed, care and treatment funds are consumed by PWAs. Fearful of the electoral consequences of conferring benefits on negatively constructed populations yet mindful of the scope of the epidemic, the deepening health-care crisis, and the inability to rationally sustain a policy which would provide treatment for women and children but not for gays or injection drug users, supporters of the act publicly focused on the benefits targeted at positively constructed groups and downplayed the obvious benefits to be received by negatively constructed populations.

The extent to which lawmakers used rhetoric to sharpen and solidify the positive construction of children with AIDS is illustrated in the House Select Committee on Children, Youth, and Families' hearing, "AIDS and Young Children in Florida," held in the year prior to passage of the Ryan White Act. Throughout the hearing, the four Congressmen present repeatedly spoke of children with AIDS as "innocent" and as "victims." In all, the Representatives used the words more than a dozen times. In contrast, none of the nine witnesses ever used these adjectives to describe children with AIDS (U.S. Congress, House, 1989). Perhaps this is a strategy on the part of the witnesses to move the social construction of PWAs away from the innocent/guilty dichotomy. In any event, the use of this rhetoric by the Congressmen is not accidental and indicates a clear intention to portray children with AIDS as a deserving population.

The House and Senate floor debate over the act provides another indication of the attempt to downplay the receipt of benefits by gays while emphasizing the benefits granted to positively constructed populations, most notably children. During the floor debate, lawmakers often relied on stories about PWAs to justify their position on the bill. Supporters of the bill told a total of nineteen such stories. Six members of Congress recounted the story of Ryan White, five told stories focusing on infants or children, three centered on women, and two on recipients of blood transfusions. Only one story included a protagonist who was identified as being gay or an IDU (both, in this case), and only one story did not reveal the context of HIV infection. This final story, though, recounted the suicide of a distraught man with AIDS who left behind a family so the sexual identity of the PWA is implicitly heterosexual. These stories are obviously not representative of the demographics of the AIDS epidemic; rather, what they reveal is the intention of policy makers to strongly emphasize the need for distributing benefits to positively constructed target populations.

The fragile rhetorical line that supporters of the bill walked was one in which they identified AIDS with sympathetic figures and alluded only elliptically to the majority of people with AIDS. Orrin Hatch, a key Republican supporter of the bill in the Senate, urged his colleagues to approve the measure by recounting the story of Tyler Spriggs, a 4-year-old with AIDS:

> I want S. 2240 for Tyler, for Belinda Mason, for Elizabeth Glaser, and her young son and for countless others, because I do not want to condemn them or any like them, regardless of who they are or what their personal lifestyles are to death. I do not care how Tyler got the disease. All I know is that he has it. I care that he get treatment. (U.S. Congress, Senate 1990a, p. S6192)

Hatch asked for tolerance for people with AIDS, but unsurprisingly chose representatives of the disease which were safe and potent symbols: heterosexual women and a young child. Though he may certainly have intended to make a broad appeal for tolerance and compassion, his choice of examples simply reinforces underlying distinctions between positively and negatively constructed groups of PWAs. Hatch's odd proclamation that "I do not care how Tyler got the disease" succeeds at once at being a self-conscious announcement of charity and a covert judgment of the majority of people with AIDS, whose behavior and "personal lifestyles" apparently make them too troublesome to explicitly mention.

But like Tyler, the late Ryan White was a useful, sympathetic symbol that lawmakers drew upon, most notably by naming the bill after him. Ryan White's death in April 1990 was widely reported in both print and electronic media and he was eulogized in each of the three major news magazines. Attaching such a potent symbol to the bill allowed its supporters to easily communicate to the public their preferred spin on legislation. Opponents of the bill understood this as well. Senator Helms saw the bill as a Trojan horse delivering benefits to gay PWAs under the guise of services to women and children. He made his feelings known: ". . . you better believe that the so-called homosexual community understood that Ryan White's story was just too good to pass up, too great an opportunity" (U.S. Congress, Senate 1990a, p. S6195).

After the bill was passed gay rights organizations hailed the law as a victory and stressed how instrumental their support for the bill had been (Castaneda, 1990), but supporters of the act never mentioned the gay lobby during debate on the bill. This is an excellent example of the sub rosa delivery of benefits to a negatively constructed target population, justified by rationales which stressed the benefits to be conferred on positively constructed populations. This interpretation is further supported by the fact that the initial draft of the bill contained a provision allowing states to waive the women and children set-asides. Thus, as originally conceived, the major substantive benefit targeted at women and children was largely symbolic. This suggests that the emphasis on "innocents with AIDS" may have been a largely rhetorical move, but during debate over the bill the waiver provision was deleted, further illustrating the connection between political language and political action.

In sum, the battle over the Ryan White CARE Act can be seen as a battle over which social constructions of the epidemic and of the people affected by the epidemic would be privileged. Supporters of the bill succeeded in crafting a version of the epidemic which emphasized its women and children "victims" and de-emphasized the extent to which benefits would be delivered to negatively constructed groups. This strategy was made possible by an expansion in the social understanding of who is at risk for HIV/AIDS, which can be traced to the 1985 Hudson/White media event. Societal learning about AIDS and the construction of multiple categories of PWAs presented a means for lawmakers to deliver benefits to a negatively constructed target population while maintaining the apparent congruence between social constructions and policy outputs in the eyes of the public. But, the rhetoric of the "innocent victim" always depended on latent images of other, guiltier PWAs to give it meaning. As I discuss below, this seemingly pragmatic rhetoric carried with it severe costs which were largely obscured in the attempt to make (some) people with AIDS into sympathetic symbols.

THE PROBLEM WITH MAKING AIDS COMFORTABLE

Though some negatively constructed groups certainly received benefits under the Ryan White Act, the problem with making AIDS comfortable in this way is the fact that lawmakers' rhetoric rein-scribed the negative images of gay men and injection drug users. At the same time it was instrumental in delivering benefits to PWAs, this rhetorical strategy failed to acknowledge the roles of key stake-holders in the AIDS policy domain. Furthermore, lawmakers uni-formly refused to challenge existing AIDS policies which actively discriminate against gay men and injection drug users although other provisions were offered and adopted which had little or nothing to do with care and treatment issues at the center of the legislation.

Foremost among the policies that went unquestioned during the Ryan White debate was the "Helms amendment." The law, introduced in 1987 by Senator Jesse Helms, prohibited the federal funding of "AIDS education, information, or prevention materials and activi-ties that promote or encourage, directly, homosexual sexual activi-ties" and it required that prevention materials emphasize "(1) absti-nence from sexual activity outside a sexually monogamous marriage (including abstinence from homosexual activities) and (2) abstinence from the use of illegal intravenous drugs" (quoted in King, 1993, p. 120). The effect of this policy, only overturned in 1992, has been to hamstring federal efforts to effectively prevent HIV infection among the population most at risk—gay men. As Edward King puts it, the Helms amendment

> reflect[s] the gulf between state-sanctioned methods of HIV prevention and those designed at the grass-roots, community level by gay men who are genuinely informed about effective means of communicating with and influencing their peers. For Helms and his colleagues, gay sex which is risk free in terms of HIV transmission is still morally lethal, and AIDS educa-tion materials which encourage safer gay sex are in fact "pro-mot[ing] sexual activity, homosexual activity . . . the very thing we want to stop." (King 1993, pp. 120-121, quote attrib-uted to Representative D. Burton)

When such a position goes fundamentally unchallenged—likely as the result of legislative compromise—and is instead combined with a political rhetoric which holds up "innocent children" as the sympa-thetic exemplars of AIDS sufferers, the de facto result for gay men is a policy of malignant neglect.

Similarly, for injection drug users, the passage of the Ryan White Act reaffirmed the prohibition on use of federal funds for the distribution of sterile needles. This provision, introduced as an amendment in the Senate, passed overwhelmingly by a vote of 98-2 amid a flurry of rhetoric about the importance of "not encouraging drug use." What such rationales obscure, though, are the ways that policies driven by stereotypes of deviance have in fact created the problem lawmakers are ostensibly interested in solving. M. Daniel Fernando (1993) argues extensively and persuasively that restrictive needle policies, including bans on access to and possession of needles, are responsible for the scarcity of clean needles, the widespread use of contaminated needles by IDUs, and thus their increased risk of HIV infection. Though the popular discourse portrays "needle sharing" as a ritual act imbedded in a drug-using subculture and thus frames the use of contaminated needles as a "choice," much of this "sharing" is actually the renting of injecting equipment by physically addicted drug users whose legal access to such equipment has been actively restricted (Fernando, 1993, pp. 75-106). Coupled with the nation's well-documented lack of drug treatment capacity, needle policies such as the one adopted with the Ryan White Act serve to exacerbate the AIDS epidemic and further reinforce the belief that HIV-positive IDUs are culpable for their sickness and beyond the help of an otherwise caring public.

The irrationality that I argue inevitably accompanies policies driven by deservedness and justified with rhetoric aimed at comforting the voting public is most obvious in the policies targeted at IDUs and children with AIDS. Lawmakers have shown considerably more concern for the plight of infected children than they have for infected IDUs and this differential concern is reflected in the way each group is treated under the Ryan White Act. The ultimate result is a policy which is self-defeating. The prevalent sense that injection drug users are deviant and undeserving and the policies such an attitude has generated have clearly hindered efforts to stem the epidemic among this group. But, not surprisingly, it has also led to increasing rates of HIV infection among their sexual partners and children. In 1985, 73% of the cases of the heterosexual transmission of HIV and 51% of the pediatric cases documented by the CDC were traceable to injection drug users (DesJarlais, Jainchill, & Friedman, 1988). A policy built on a negative construction of injection drug users has had the serious consequence of inhibiting efforts to reduce the rates of infection among the ostensibly more deserving populations of women and children—populations which were publicly held up by lawmakers as the compelling rationale for passing the law in the first place.

The discourse about AIDS in the United States has certainly changed over time, and the most popular account holds that after an initial bout of misplaced prejudice the American public learned about AIDS and accepted the message that "everyone is at risk." The mass media produced messages generalizing the fear of AIDS (such as the July 1985 cover of *Life* which proclaimed "NOW NO ONE IS SAFE FROM AIDS"), and Americans came to understand that non-drug injecting heterosexuals and children could be infected with HIV. But in the rush to increase public acceptance of people with AIDS and spur a reluctant government into action, activists and lawmakers promoted a version of the epidemic which focused on its most sympathetic sufferers and quietly pushed the less sympathetic majority out of sight.

The debate over the Ryan White Act is the exemplary illustration of how this strategy operated, but it also shows its shortcomings. Because legislators used rationales based on deservedness, they could not erase—and in the end perhaps only highlighted—the perception that other groups were undeserving. Gay men and injection drug users, in particular, were effectively omitted from the Ryan White Act debate except when the lawmakers seemed driven to reinforce their deviance through punitive provisions. They were certainly not given a voice and were not directly represented either in the statements of lawmakers or through any of the letters or statements members of Congress included in the *Congressional Record.*

CONCLUSION

At first glance, one might praise the more progressive lawmakers who championed the Ryan White Act for devising a clever rhetorical strategy which allowed a legislative compromise. Even though the Act had yet to be fully funded by 1994, the provision of any treatment funds must be welcomed, especially in the face of an overburdened, unreformed health care system. But I contend that this important, partial, short-term gain was purchased at considerable risk. Having at least symbolically taken care of the "most deserving" people with AIDS, the risk is that the "less deserving" will continue to slip through the very wide cracks of the country's health care system in ever increasing numbers.

While the number of people with AIDS continues to grow, the rhetoric of innocence increasingly rings hollow. But however empty, this rhetoric is still loud enough to drown out the voices of the majority of people with AIDS. In 1993, the most recent year for which information is available, the largest group of new AIDS cases was still gay men who, together with injection drug users, accounted for 77% of all new cases (CDC, 1994, p. 8).[5] But, trends in new HIV infections show a changing profile of the epidemic, and these changes can only be expected to heighten the marginalization of people with AIDS. According to the CDC, nearly three quarters of the new HIV infections in 1994 were among drug users, an increasing number of them crack users (Kolata, 1995). Thus, as gay men remain the largest population of PWAs, the epidemic continues to dig deeper into the inner city, affecting disproportionate numbers of women, members of minority groups, drug addicts, and the poor—populations which to this point have been largely politically powerless.

Even as the demographic trends of the epidemic shift, the political rhetoric about people with AIDS remains the same. In his first major address on AIDS policy, Bill Clinton noted that "I have a friend who lost her mother and another friend who lost his wife to AIDS because of tainted blood transfusion, and many others" ("Excerpts from President's Speech," 1993). Although he undoubtedly intended this line to show his personal connection with the issue, it is difficult not to miss the fact that President Clinton confined his personal association with AIDS to "innocent victims." Such rhetoric may be guided by the belief that sympathy for the "innocent" is readily transferable to those unmentioned, who are, perhaps, a bit more "guilty." But it is not sympathy that is needed. What is needed in the United States is political leadership which unflinchingly confronts the AIDS epidemic as a crisis which confronts citizens—not cuddly children, perverted homosexuals, or dirty drug addicts—but *citizens* who have a stake and should have a voice in the policies which affect their lives.

With a tide of political conservatism apparently sweeping the country there seems a fair chance that the political scripts of denial and blame may very well be revived in the discourse about AIDS. Indeed the battle over the reauthorization of the Ryan White Act may provide a forum for just such a spectacle. Such rhetoric has already surfaced in the increasingly moralistic debate over welfare reform. But even if this does not happen, the challenge to activists will certainly not disappear: While there are no clear strategies for success, it is vitally important not to misrepresent the character of the crisis. Pushing already marginalized citizens into the shadows in order to win them political favors may result in short-term gains— and certainly we should be careful about casually dismissing such gains in a crisis as pressing as the AIDS epidemic. But while allur- ing, "Trojan horse" strategies intended to smuggle the concerns of negatively constructed groups into the policy debate are fatally flawed. Such strategies fail to acknowledge—and in fact deny—that such groups are legitimate stakeholders, and result in already disen- franchised citizens being left dependent on political generosity which is rarely forthcoming.

NOTES

1. Hughes (1993) presents a similar, though slightly different paradigm.

2. I have focused on Ryan White because his story was so prominent, but there were other children with AIDS whose stories were key to reframing the image of PWAs. The Ray brothers of Arcadia, Florida, for example, were the subject of network news coverage when they were excluded from school and driven out of town by an arson-fire which destroyed their home. See David L. Kirp's book *Learning by Heart: AIDS and Schoolchildren in America's Communities* and Robin Nagle's chapter in James Kinsella's (1989) *Covering the Plague.*

3. This section is adapted from my earlier article "The Social Constructions of People with AIDS: Target Populations and United States Policy, 1981-1990" (Donovan, 1993).

4. The arrangement of groups in Figure 1 is based primarily on the informed perceptions of the author, but should have face validity to those familiar with the history of HIV/AIDS in the United States. The placement of the most "deviant" groups should make sense to those simply familiar with the prevailing American

conceptions of drug use and homosexuality. Each of the groups listed in Figure 1 is discussed as an identifiable group in a wide variety of commentary on the AIDS epidemic (in addition to those cited in the body of the text, the following sources were also consulted: Bayer, 1989; Crimp, 1988; Epstein, 1991; Grmek, 1990; Hallet, 1994; Hughey, Norton, & Sullivan-Norton, 1989; MacKinnon, 1992; Presidential Commission on the Human Immunodeficiency Virus Epidemic, 1988; Price, 1992; Quam & Ford, 1990; Ron & Rogers, 1989; Wachter, 1992). Additionally, the CDC classifies adult AIDS cases (kept distinct from pediatric cases) as falling into "exposure categories" which reinforces the distinction of these separate target populations: "men who have sex with men," "injecting drug use," "men who have sex with men and inject drugs," "hemophilia/coagulation disorder," "heterosexual contact," and "receipt of blood transfusion, blood components, or tissue." From a policy design perspective, the Ryan White Act specifically targets provisions at women, children, and hemophiliacs (Title II), blood transfusion recipients (Title III), and injection drug users (Titles II, III, and IV[Subtitle C]). Furthermore, each of the groups listed in Figure 1 is represented politically by activist and advocacy groups such as the AIDS Coalition to Unleash Power (ACT-UP), Gay Men's Health Crisis, The National Hemophilia Foundation, Pediatric AIDS Coalition, and the PWA Coalition (which supports an International Working Group on Women and AIDS).

5. According to the most recent data from the CDC, the number of new AIDS cases dropped slightly from 85,944 in 1992-93 to 85,260 in 1993-94. People fitting into the exposure categories "men who have sex with men," "injecting drug use," and "men who have sex with men and inject drugs" accounted for 81.9% of new AIDS cases in 1992-93 (70,405 cases), and 77.1% of new AIDS cases in 1993-94 (65,737 cases). In contrast, 822 cases of pediatric AIDS were diagnosed in 1992-93 and 992 cases were diagnosed in 1993-94 (CDC, 1994, p. 8).

REFERENCES

Albert, E. (1989). AIDS and the press: The creation and transformation of a social problem. In Joel Best (Ed.), *Images of issues: Typifying contemporary social problems* (pp. 39-54). New York: Aldine de Gruyter.

Altman, D. (1986). *AIDS in the mind of America*. New York: Anchor Press/Doubleday.

Bayer, R. (1989). *Private acts, social consequences: AIDS and the politics of public health*. New York: The Free Press.

Brandt, A. M. (1985). *No magic bullet: A social history of venereal disease in the United States since 1880*. New York: Oxford University Press.

Brandt, A. M. (1988). AIDS: From social history to social policy. In E. Fee & D. M. Fox (Eds.), *AIDS: The burdens of history* (pp. 147-171). Berkeley: University of California Press.

Brandt, A. M. (1991). AIDS and metaphor: Toward the social meaning of epidemic disease. In A. Mack (Ed.), *In time of plague: The history and social consequences of lethal epidemic disease* (pp. 91-110). New York: New York University Press.

Castaneda, Ruben. (1990). Gay rights fund-raiser marks gains; Group cites 3 progressive bills, ties with hill, White House. *Washington Post*, 7 October, B3 (Metro). Lexis text retrieval.

Centers for Disease Control and Prevention. (1994). *HIV/AIDS Surveillance Report*, 6:1.

Congressional Quarterly Almanac. (1990). Washington DC: Congressional Quarterly, Inc.

Cook, T. E., & D. C. Colby. (1992). The mass-mediated epidemic. In E. Fee & D. M. Fox (Eds.), *AIDS: The making of a chronic disease* (pp. 84-122). Berkeley: University of California Press.

Corea, G. (1992). *The invisible epidemic: The story of women and AIDS*. New York: HarperCollins.

Crimp, D. (Ed.). (1988). *AIDS: Cultural analysis/cultural activism*. Boston: MIT Press.

Dery, D. (1984). *Problem definition in policy analysis*. Lawrence: University of Kansas Press.

Des Jarlais, D. C., Jainchill, N., & Friedman, S. R. (1988). AIDS among IV drug users: Epidemiology, natural history, and therapeutic community experiences. In R. Galea, B. Lewis, & L. Baker (Eds.), *AIDS and IV drug users* (pp. 51-59). Owings Mills, MD: National Health Publishing.

Donovan, M. C. (1993). The social constructions of people with AIDS: Target populations and United States policy, 1981-1990. *Policy Studies Review, 12*(3/4), 3-29.

Epstein, S. (1991). Democratic science? AIDS activism and the contested construction of knowledge. *Socialist Review, 21*(April-June), 35-64.

Excerpts from president's speech on AIDS research efforts. (1993, December 2). *New York Times*, p. A12.

Fee, E. (1988). Sin versus science: Venereal disease in twentieth-century Baltimore. In E. Fee & D. M. Fox (Eds.), *AIDS: The burdens of history* (pp. 121-146). Berkeley: University of California Press.

Fernando, M. D. (1993). *AIDS and intravenous drug use: The influence of morality, politics, social science, and race in the making of a tragedy*. Westport, CT: Praeger.

Galea, R., B. Lewis, & L. Baker (Eds.). (1988). AIDS and IV drug users. Owings Mills, MD: National Health Publishing.

Gilman, S. L. (1988). *Disease and representation: Images of illness from madness to AIDS*. Ithaca: Cornell University Press.

Grmek, M. D. (1990). *History of AIDS: Emergence and origin of a modern pandemic*. (Russell C. Maulitz & Jacalyn Duffin, Trans.). Princeton: Princeton University Press.

Hallett, M. A., & D. Cannella. (1994). Gatekeeping through Media format: Strategies of voice for the HIV-positive via human interest news formats and organization. *Journal of Homosexuality, 26*(4), 111-134.

Hughes, C. G. (1993). The piper's dance: A paradigm of the collective response to epidemic disease. *International Journal of Mass Emergencies and Disasters, 11*(August), 227-245.

Hughey, J. D., R. W. Norton, & C. Sullivan-Norton. (1989). Insidious metaphors and the changing meaning of AIDS. *AIDS & Public Policy Journal, 4*(spring), 56-67.

King, E. (1993). *Safety in numbers: Safer sex and gay men.* New York: Routledge.

Kinsella, J. (1989). *Covering the plague: AIDS and the American media.* New Brunswick: Rutgers University Press.

Kirp, David L., with S. Epstein et al. (1989). *Learning by heart: AIDS and schoolchildren in America's communities.* New Brunswick: Rutgers University Press.

Kolata, G. (1995, February 28). New picture of who will get AIDS is crammed with addicts. *New York Times*, p. B6.

MacKinnon, K. (1992). *The politics of popular representation: Reagan, Thatcher, AIDS, and the movies.* Cranbury, NJ: Associated University Press.

Nagle, R. (1989). A plague in the villages. In James Kinsella, *Covering the plague: AIDS and the American media* (pp. 185-209). New Brunswick: Rutgers University Press.

National Research Council. (1993). *The social impact of AIDS in the United States.* Washington, DC: National Academy Press.

National Research Council. (1990). *AIDS: The second decade.* Washington, DC: National Academy Press.

Nelkin, D., & S. L. Gilman. (1991). Placing blame for devastating disease. In A. Mack (Ed.), *In time of plague: The history and social consequences of lethal epidemic disease* (pp. 39-56). New York: New York University Press.

Patton, C. (1990). *Inventing AIDS.* New York: Routledge.

Presidential Commission on the Human Immunodeficiency Virus Epidemic. (1988). *Report of the Presidential Commission on the Human Immunodeficiency Virus Epidemic.* Washington, DC: Government Printing Office.

Price, C. (1992). AIDS, organization of drug users, and public policy. *AIDS & Public Policy Journal, 7*, 141-144.

Quam, M., & N. Ford. (1990). AIDS policies and practices in the United States. In B. Misztal & D. Moss (Eds.), *Action on AIDS: National policies in comparative perspective* (pp. 25-50). New York: Greenwood Press.

Rogers, E. M., J. W. Dearing, & S. Chang. (1991). AIDS in the 1980s: The agenda-setting process for a public issue. *Journalism Monographs*, No. 126. Association for Education in Journalism and Mass Communication.

Ron, A., & D. E. Rogers. (1989). AIDS in the United States: Patient care and politics. *Daedalus, 118*(2), 41-58.

Rosenberg, C. (1989). What is an epidemic? AIDS in historical perspective. *Daedalus, 118*(2), 1-17.

Ryan White Comprehensive AIDS Resources Emergency Act of 1990. (1990). U.S. code (P.L. 101-381).

Schneider, A., & H. Ingram. (1993). The social construction of target populations:

Implications for politics and policy. *American Political Science Review, 87,* 334-347.

Shilts, Randy. (1987). *And the band played on: Politics, people, and the AIDS epidemic.* New York: Penguin Books.

Treichler, P. A. (1988). AIDS, gender, and biomedical discourse. In E. Fee & D. M. Fox (Eds.), *AIDS: The burdens of history* (pp. 190-266). Berkeley: University of California Press.

U.S. Congress. House. (1989). Select Committee on Children, Youth, and Families. *AIDS and young children in south Florida.* 101st Congress, 1st Session, 7 August.

U.S. Congress. Senate. (1990a). 101st Congress, 2nd Session. *Congressional record* (15 May), vol. 136, pt. 1.

U.S. Congress. Senate. (1990b). 101st Congress, 2nd Session. *Congressional record* (16 May), vol. 136, pt. 1.

Wachter, R. M. (1992). AIDS, activism, and the politics of health. *The New England Journal of Medicine* (January 9), 128-133.

A Citizens' AIDS Task Force:
Overcoming Obstacles

Jane Harris Aiken, JD, LLM

University of South Carolina

SUMMARY. This article analyzes the experience of a state-wide Task Force on AIDS using grassroots techniques to construct policy responsive to the needs of people living with HIV. The four primary obstacles to effective policy making were the need (1) to include disenfranchised groups; (2) to avoid the domination of governmental bureaucracy so that community-based organizations could offer solutions, as well as services; (3) to overcome resistance to anonymous testing; and (4) to reach "hard to reach" populations. Task Force members' perspectives colored what were deemed appropriate policies. Members tended to polarize into two groups: those community-based groups and individuals who focused on the needs of people with HIV on one side, and on the other side, more institutional players who wanted to identify and isolate "HIV carriers." The article closes by analyzing the resulting HIV Omnibus Bill. Those who focused on the needs of people with HIV seized the opportunity to

Jane Harris Aiken is Professor of Law at the University of South Carolina and is Coordinator of the Women and HIV Law Project of USC's pro bono program. She was the chair of the Arizona Governor's Task Force on AIDS from 1988 to 1990 and the former Director of Arizona State University's HIV Legal Clinic.

The author would like to thank Catherine Smith for her excellent assistance in preparing this article.

Correspondence may be addressed: School of Law, The University of South Carolina, Columbia, SC 29208.

[Haworth co-indexing entry note]: "A Citizens' AIDS Task Force: Overcoming Obstacles." Aiken, Jane Harris. Co-published simultaneously in *Journal of Homosexuality* (The Haworth Press, Inc.) Vol. 32, No. 3/4, 1997, pp. 145-167; and: *Activism and Marginalization in the AIDS Crisis* (ed: Michael A. Hallett) The Haworth Press, Inc., 1997, pp. 145-167; and: *Activism and Marginalization in the AIDS Crisis* (ed: Michael A. Hallett) Harrington Park Press, an imprint of The Haworth Press, Inc., 1997, pp. 145-167. Single or multiple copies of this article are available for a fee from The Haworth Document Delivery Service [1-800-342-9678, 9:00 a.m. - 5:00 p.m. (EST). E-mail address: get info@haworth.com].

145

draft and successfully pass an omnibus bill through the Arizona Legislature. This success demonstrates that highly organized communities can affect policy making, even to the extent that it offsets more institutionalized power. *[Article copies available for a fee from The Haworth Document Delivery Service: 1-800-342-9678. E-mail address: getinfo@haworth.com]*

Dana Mims[1] went to his doctor for some routine, not HIV related, care. The doctor discussed his HIV condition in front of the nurse receptionist. The nurse recognized the man as a produce worker at her local grocery store. That evening, she talked to the store manager and told him that she did not want to buy produce handled by a person with AIDS. The grocery store fired him the next day. A local television station learned of his predicament and offered him a chance to tell his story on a local news show. He agreed and they presented it, with his real name and shadowed face. That evening, the landlord evicted him from his apartment. His father, after whom he was named, called to tell him that he never wanted to see him again. Apparently, many people had seen the story and recognized the name. People believed that his father had AIDS and shunned him. The father's response was to distance himself from his namesake. At the time, there was little legal recourse for this man. His life was in a shambles. The disease did not cause these problems. The reaction to it did. He was not alone. He had found many others who had had similar experiences. In 1987, the Americans with Disabilities Act did not exist and there was little that the law could do to protect someone identified as HIV-positive.

In 1987, the Governor of Arizona recommended more punitive sodomy laws as a solution to the HIV epidemic. Advocates for people with HIV/AIDS remained silent in the face of the health crisis for fear that the Governor would enact oppressive and homophobic policies. The Governor, through his hateful policies and alleged misuse of campaign funds, created concern among more than the AIDS activist community. The legislature impeached him. The Secretary of State, Rose Mofford, became Governor. Governor Mofford established a Governor's Task Force on AIDS as one of her first executive acts. Arizona now joined states all over the nation that had established Task Forces to develop strategies for surviving this national epidemic.

This was the year that Randy Shilts published *And the Band Played On* documenting how the United States government had turned a blind eye to HIV for many years while more people succumbed to the disease (Shilts, 1987). Only after the press began to report stories of HIV in the heterosexual population did the disease begin to receive mainstream attention. Governmental entities rarely call on professionals to deliver vital services until a crisis compels them to take emergency action and such was the case in Arizona. The Governor created the Task Force after Arizona was well into an epidemic. Arizona citizens were frightened and people with HIV were struggling to survive with little or no help from the government. Arizona, like the rest of the nation, was dealing with the large federal cutbacks in poverty programs, housing, health care, and social services.

THE GOAL

Since Arizona was late in the process of dealing with HIV, the task was staggering. High energy and fresh ideas were essential. The Task Force was a mission-driven organization while the Public Health Department was a rule-driven bureaucratic organization. Mission-driven organizations tend to be more efficient and effective. They are more innovative and flexible than rule-driven organizations. Mission-driven organizations also have a higher morale than rule-driven organizations (Osborne & Gaebler, 1993, pp. 117-133).

The Governor defined the mission of the Task Force:

- Identify means to curb the spread of HIV/AIDS;
- Create systems of care for persons with HIV/AIDS;
- Develop policies for addressing the HIV epidemic in Arizona.[2]

We believed as a central premise that compassionate care and treatment of people with HIV would prevent further spread of HIV/AIDS. The Task Force was formed at a time when public officials were pitting the civil rights of people with AIDS against the rights of the uninfected. Our belief was that there was no tension between civil rights and public health. Unless we protect the civil liberties of people with HIV, there can be no public health. People who were afraid of discrimination had no incentive to know their HIV status nor to identify themselves so that they could be counseled about safer sex and receive appropriate treatment. We wanted to create policies that met the needs of Arizona citizens at risk for AIDS rather than catering to the fears and stereotypes of people who sought to repress people with HIV. We were faced with four obstacles: trying to include disenfranchised groups in our decision-making process; focusing on a community effort unhampered by the bureaucracy of government; ensuring anonymous testing; and representing "hard to reach populations."

OBSTACLE 1:
INCLUSION OF DISENFRANCHISED GROUPS

Our first obstacle was to ensure that people with HIV played a significant role in the direction of the Task Force. The 45 members of the Task Force came from many parts of the community: grass-roots organizations, the police and fire departments, public health departments, the state legislature, religious organizations, and the business and health care community. The Governor's office chose the members after soliciting the community for names of people who had been active in HIV issues. They culled the names to ensure that the group would be acceptable to the public, veering away from activists. Despite my work advocating the rights of people with HIV, I was chosen as chair largely, I believe, because as an academic, people perceived me as "neutral" and therefore acceptable. Despite the culling, all of the Task Force members came with their own agendas. It would only be a matter of time before we discovered each agenda.

The Task Force was not truly representative. Only one member of the Task Force identified himself as HIV-positive although many community groups providing care and services to HIV-positive individuals were official members. The HIV community criticized the Governor for her failure to include more people with HIV on the Task Force. The lack of people with HIV causes more than political problems. People with HIV focus on their capacities rather than their deficiencies. That stance can make a great deal of difference when drafting policy. We wanted policies that allowed people to live with the disease not be victimized by it.

The Task Force lacked racial diversity. Only two members were African American, four were Latinos, and one was Pima Indian. The Navajo nation occupies a large portion of the state of Arizona. Despite a rising incidence of HIV on the reservation, there were no Navajo members on the Task Force. Although many Task Force members were gay, only one member publicly identified himself as gay. This was particularly troubling since at the time of the Task Force's inception, over 75% of the known cases of HIV in the state were within the gay population.

In 1987, nationally we were beginning to see that people of color were disproportionately affected by HIV. In Arizona, the vast majority of the AIDS cases were attributable to homosexual contact. People assumed that that meant white gay men. Indeed white gay men had been in the forefront in Arizona in educating about the disease. The Health Department's statistics indicated that whites accounted for 86% of all AIDS cases, a figure higher than their proportion in Arizona's population (75%). Most of the Health Department's efforts were directed toward the white community. Even though a large number of the cases were among white gay men, the national figures revealed that by 1990, members of minority groups made up 43 percent of all AIDS cases attributed to unprotected homosexual contact (Sills, 1994, p. 66).[3]

Being a member of the Task Force was somewhat of a thankless job, unpaid, and with a charge that could have kept the 45 people appointed to the Task Force busy full-time for the year. To solve the work load and the diversity needs, members were eager to chair subcommittees of nonappointed members who were interested in particular subjects. This expanded our active membership into approximately 250 people. Many of the nonappointed members were people with HIV or people who worked closely with people with HIV in grass-roots community organizations. As the year of study progressed, we focused attention on the concerns of Latinos, African Americans, and Native Americans and added more representatives of color to our membership. The large numbers appear cumbersome. However, we identified specific issues of concern and assigned committees to develop particular policies in those areas. Because each committee's charge was manageable, the larger group accomplished things that the 45-body unit could not effectively do. Because the subcommittees included many people with HIV, they generated policies more sensitive to their needs. We became more representative of people with HIV and people of color using nonappointed members in this committee structure. However, this structure presented a new obstacle: how to sell the product to the larger (less representative) body?

OBSTACLE 2: BUREAUCRACY vs. COMMUNITY

The Public Health Department housed the Task Force. From the beginning of the Task Force work, there were turf battles with public health officials. In many states, Task Forces were initiated out of the Public Health Department. This Task Force, instead, had been initiated as a citizens' Task Force with the obligation to report to the Governor. The Health Department was to play a role but not direct the course of investigation. The hope was that the Task Force would develop policies free of bureaucratic restraints.

Public health has generally been a friend to people with HIV as the epidemic has progressed. Medical associations have often pushed for exclusionary and oppressive policies when dealing with HIV. Public health has offered more reasoned responses to calls for repressive acts against people with HIV (Fox, 1988). Nevertheless, a public health department, like any bureaucracy, prefers to establish its own policy and not be hamstrung by citizen advisory groups charged with establishing policy.

Community-based organizations provided much of the care for people with HIV. They relied upon volunteers and charitable donations to survive. Although those groups were extremely effective in the delivery of services, it was unconscionable that in the face of a serious health crisis, the State was abandoning citizens' needs to charity. At the time I did not understand that pulling ownership of services out of the community and into the government weakens the community and undermines the people (Osborne & Gaebler, 1993).[4] As the Task Force work progressed, this lesson became more apparent. We sought to use government to promote policies that would be supportive of community efforts to provide care for people with HIV.

There are significant differences between a community approach to policy and the bureaucratic approach of the Public Health Department. As Osborne and Gaebler (1993) have noted, communities have more commitment to their members than service delivery systems have to their clients. They understand their members' problems better than service professionals. Institutions offer "service"; communities offer "care." They provide that care in much more creative and flexible ways. Our challenge as a Task Force was to create policies that vested communities with the service delivery while dealing with the public health need for bureaucratic control.

HIV prevention programs received the bulk of their funding from the federal government. The state of Arizona was devoting precious few resources to HIV health issues. Therefore, the Public Health Department needed to establish that Arizona deserved to receive a large percentage of the funds that were available nationally. In 1988, Arizona ranked 22nd in the nation for the number of reported HIV cases. The case rate per 100,000 in 1987 indicated that Arizona's cases were growing at the same rate as Illinois, which ranked seventh in the nation.

Drug smugglers used Arizona's Indian reservations as a drug corridor from Mexico. Smugglers could get well into the United States largely avoiding state highways patrolled by state police. Drug couriers from Mexico would enter Arizona through the reservation and seek harbor with desperately poor Native Americans. Often the drug dealers paid for such services in drugs. Needles were shared. Therefore the authorities thought that the incidence of HIV caused by needle sharing and heterosexual activity on the reservation was fairly high, although the numbers were not available.

Arizona attracted people with HIV. The desert climate was appealing. Phoenix and Tucson had well-developed AIDS service organizations and the University of Arizona was a site for HIV drug experimentation through the National Institutes of Health. Some of the most important, cutting-edge drug experimentation for HIV/AIDS occurred at the University of Arizona. This made Arizona an attractive place to move to for people in Los Angeles who were dealing with overwhelmed HIV/AIDS service organizations and inadequate treatment facilities. Many people with HIV had moved to Arizona after their diagnosis. Their numbers were also difficult to ascertain. The health department maintained that the number of people in Arizona infected with HIV was much higher than the "official" number reported. Community groups documented their needs for funds through the number of people served. The Health Department sought to demonstrate the need for funds through confirmed names of persons tested positive for HIV. This bureaucratic approach reduced people to numbers and characterized much of the mainstream perception of public health.

Relations with the Public Health Department, the body most likely to carry out any recommendations of the Task Force were cool. This antagonism between the Health Department and the community to be served prompted many of the people working on and with the Task Force to push for legislation so that policies recommended by the Task Force would have the force of law and not be subject to administrative discretion.

OBSTACLE 3: ANONYMOUS TESTING

One of the critical issues for people with HIV was anonymous testing and avoiding by-name reporting of HIV-positive status (Bayer, Levine, & Wolf, 1991). Since the University of Arizona was a site for experimental drug testing in the HIV area, early detection could allow one to qualify for new and possibly effective drugs. People were eager to know their status but concerned that unless they had anonymous tests, they would face substantial discrimination in employment and insurance, and rejection by family and friends. The community was well aware of many examples of discrimination. Landlords and families had thrown people out of their homes. Employers had fired people from their jobs. Doctors were surreptitiously testing and refused to treat patients who tested positive for HIV. Insurance companies canceled insurance or raised their premiums beyond reach when they discovered a patient's HIV-positive status.

Working groups asked people to come forward and tell their stories.[5] Joe Wentworth,[6] a music teacher at a local elementary school, told of the medical resident who came into his hospital room while his boss was visiting. The resident, clad from head to toe in green scrubs, a surgical mask, gloves, and goggles, interrupted the conversation to ask Joe how he had gotten AIDS. The boss, unaware of the diagnosis, fled the hospital room. Upon release from the hospital, Joe found that he no longer had a job.

Another person sadly told of the suicide of his lover. While he had been in the hospital with an unexplained illness, the hospital tested him for HIV and found him to be positive. A doctor went to the visiting room and reported the positive test results to the lover, noting that he might be better able to communicate the news to his friend. Convinced that he was infected as well, the lover jumped to his death from the window of the hospital. The autopsy revealed that he tested negative for the virus. No one had bothered to counsel him about his risk.

We consistently heard of breaches in the Health Department's promise of confidentiality in their lists of HIV-infected people. This included allegations that the Department routinely gave the names to the police department. During our deliberation, the *Arizona Republic* newspaper reported that the Phoenix police kept lists of people suspected to be HIV-positive in their police car computer. Some people with HIV alleged that when they called the police or emergency vehicles, they were slow to respond or failed to come at all. They attributed this failure to their identification through the Health Department. The police chief confirmed the list but declined to tell where the department had gotten the names.

A physician told the working group that to refrain from reporting a person by name to the Health Department, he routinely avoided using HIV tests but monitored the person's T-cell count. This procedure was much more expensive. However, this method kept him in compliance with regulations. The regulation did not require reporting the names of persons with HIV/AIDS but merely those who tested positive for HIV. He had found that once a person tested positive for HIV, insurance companies were reluctant to pay for services and eventually would terminate coverage or raise the premiums so high that the person could not afford the health insurance. His strategies, however, were beginning to fail. He had been identified as an "AIDS doc" by the Health Department and insurance companies. This identity subjected him to Health Department drop-in checks of his records (as allowed by state law) and more rigorous scrutiny and paperwork requirements from insurance companies. Carrying the load of most of the HIV cases in Phoenix was stressful enough without the interference of the State and insurance industry.

A surgeon urged the Task Force to allow him to test any patient who came to him for medical treatment. He argued that he, his family, and staff should not be put at risk of infection when it was very easy to know who was infected with the virus. Once he knew the HIV status of the patient, then he could decide if he wanted to encounter the risk the patient posed. If he should choose to operate, then he could warn the operating staff and use appropriate precautions. He exhorted the Task Force to allow testing for the protection of all health care workers and access to Health Department lists of persons known to be HIV-infected.

Temporarily, anonymous testing and counseling were available through county health departments. If a private facility tested the individual and determined he was infected, the tester reported the person by name to the health department. In rural communities, a visit to the county health department for an "anonymous test" was tantamount to announcing one was HIV-infected. Public authorities resisted anonymous testing and urged by-name reporting of HIV status to document the rate of infection in Arizona. Those numbers had a great impact on the amount of money appropriated to Arizona from the federal government.

The Task Force investigated the issue. At a public forum, the Health Department's head epidemiologist argued for by-name reporting, stating the need for more accurate statistics on the incidence of HIV in Arizona. A lawyer for an HIV-positive advocacy group presented the arguments for anonymous testing. She recounted many of the stories that the work group had heard. The Health Department resented being second guessed about this issue. Throughout the process they resisted efforts by the Task Force to require making some form of anonymous testing available.

We eventually recommended that anonymous testing be available at county health department test sites. We also recommended that the Health Department certify physicians and other health care providers to do anonymous testing and counseling. Such certified physicians would be exempt from reporting HIV-positive status by the name of the client. They merely needed to report the total number of those testing HIV-positive.[7]

OBSTACLE 4:
REACHING THE "HARD TO REACH" POPULATIONS

Rural Areas

Phoenix was headquarters for the Task Force with many members from Tucson. Thus, the urban areas within Arizona were well represented. Determining the needs of people in rural areas and on reservations was a challenge. One possible avenue for getting information from those areas was to use the local health departments as resources. Given the concerns and partial distrust with the public health community, we were unsure whether this was a good source for determining the true concerns of people with HIV. One way to reach remote populations was to gain some access through gay groups within the rural areas. We used our contacts in the gay community to try to get in touch with people in outlying areas to identify what the needs were for people with HIV. This worked only to a degree. Rural gays were at risk for stigmatization if they were identified as gay and, particularly, if the community knew they had HIV/AIDS. We needed to make it safe to discuss the issue without being identified. Our partial solution to this problem was to make sure that we went to every area of the state and held "hearings" at a local community center.

The hearings included formal presentations about the Task Force's work. We took testimony from local citizens who had concerns about how the state was dealing with HIV. We also made sure that we were available informally both before and after the public forum. We held twenty-one of these public meetings. We made sure that when the Task Force was "on the road" in rural areas, we had a representative group. I went as the Chair, a white woman, but we also had representatives from the Black, Latino, Native American, and gay communities. These meetings sometimes erupted into discussions about how Arizona was doing little to nothing about the health and treatment needs in their communities. We found that there were precious few opportunities in which the government came to them for input into what policies they needed and wanted carried out. Understandably, the frustration and the concerns were far greater than the issue of HIV. Thus the public hearings were often heated. People who testified offered example after example of the State's indifference to their needs. This resulted in fairly negative press for the State and the Task Force. One headline in the Tucson paper suggested that the Task Force itself was indifferent to the needs of people of color. This article stemmed from efforts to gain input from local minority groups. A reporter present at the meeting noted the overt distrust of government demonstrated by the people testifying. The inclusion of the Task Force in this distrust was fostered by our attempts to validate their experience. Such validation was intended to signal our receptiveness but was interpreted by the press as confirmation.[8] The negatives were short-lived but the contacts were significant. These meetings energized new people into the effort to define the HIV policy. The meetings brought together many people with similar agendas. Gay people of color had been abandoned by the government, the churches in their communities, and the predominately white HIV service community. These hearings offered opportunities for these groups to come together and be heard. Their problems were complex due to the intersection of racism and heterosexism. However, the meetings emphasized the commonalities and generated new energy for solutions. Many of those people are still working together on larger health issues at the grassroots level (Briathwaite, 1991, p. 522).

Native American Reservations

On reservations, the problems of reaching people were even more complex. These were people accustomed to being ignored and abused by the State of Arizona. Since the Task Force was an organization of government, the people treated us with suspicion. We held public hearings for the Pima, Havasupi, Navajo, Apache, and Hopi Indians. There were very few gay-identified groups within the Native American population. Although there was some sexual activity between persons of the same sex, there was generally no "gay-identified" identity culturally. Therefore, our strategy of reaching the gay community to avoid relying solely on the Health Department did not work in Indian country. We tried to make connections while at the public hearings and we recruited as many Native Americans into our subcommittees as we could find. We tried to make the needs of Native Americans an explicit concern addressed by each subject matter group. The Task Force ultimately failed to deal adequately with issues that arise for Native Americans in Arizona. This was largely due to our failure to follow through with ideas that arose in the Native American communities. Our excuse was that we felt incompetent to deal with the complex jurisdictional issues that policy making for Native Americans entailed. As a state governmental body, we were reluctant to suggest policy for independent nations. However, upon analysis, Indian people were largely disenfranchised in the process. Jurisdiction really was a red herring: it was easier to avoid dealing with the complex problems. There were few Native Americans represented on the Task Force and the non-Indian population ignored the stated needs of Native American people. The structural interests of Native American people did not "fit" within the basic logic and principles by which the public health system operated. There were no social or political institutions that ensured that these interests were served. The Task Force contributed to the repression of these interests. Alford (1975) suggests that in order for such repressed structural interests to be heard, enormous political and organizational energies must be summoned to offset the intrinsic disadvantages of the position. Given the overwhelming problems facing native peoples in Arizona, the issue of HIV was not a top priority worthy of the kind of effort that might have created policy initiatives useful to Indian people.

TAKING ACTION:
SECURING RIGHTS vs. SECURING RISKS

After almost a year of collecting information and identifying needs for people with HIV, the group set about the task of drafting recommendations. Each group identified the issues that arose in their subject matter areas and drafted proposed recommendations. We used a standard format: each recommendation included an issue statement, a section that described the background of the issue, a recommendation of the Task Force, and an implementation strategy.[9] For example, one issue was "Should anonymous testing and counseling be available on a more widespread basis?" The background section detailed the availability of anonymous testing in Arizona, the limitations of county health sites, the position of the health department, and the benefits of testing and counseling for people who suspect that they may be HIV-positive. The background also documented some studies that indicated that less people are willing to be tested if testing is not anonymous. After that background section, the Task Force made three recommendations:

- Expand anonymous testing to nongovernmental sites;
- Create a certification process for physicians who wish to test so that they will do effective and compassionate counseling;
- Clarify that persons tested at anonymous sites and by certified physicians need not be reported by name.

The implementation section suggested that this be done through legislation and administrative rule making.

We needed to develop approximately fifty different issues along this format. Almost immediately, we became polarized. At one end of the spectrum were the people who focused on the needs of people with HIV and viewed their role as securing rights. On the other end of the spectrum were those who wanted to identify and isolate "HIV carriers." Those focused on the needs of people with HIV included community-based care providers, people living with HIV, civil libertarians, and people who had had enough contact with people with HIV to have developed an understanding and compassionate approach to their needs. This group identified their concerns as fashioning some civil rights protection for people with HIV against discrimination in services, housing, and employment. They sought criminal penalties and damage actions for breach of confidentiality by individuals who gained access to HIV-sensitive information. Many members of this group urged protection for people with HIV from discrimination in health insurance. An overriding concern was ensuring affordable and effective health care for people through every stage of the illness. They also urged comprehensive age-appropriate HIV/AIDS education for all school children and HIV education for all state employees likely to have contact with people with HIV. The group challenged the current practice of the

Health Department to clear all HIV education materials through a community board to decide if the brochures were "offensive."[10] They urged more outreach to the gay community. Finally, this group pushed for the State to substantially increase the resources directed toward HIV. The Task Force urged the State to put those resources into providing health care and subsidizing access to effective drugs rather than contact tracing and epidemiological studies.

At the polar extreme were those people who perceived others as risk creators and their role as policy makers was to secure risks. National public health figures facilitated this by the early use of the term "risk groups." This characterization suggests that membership in a particular group causes HIV rather than individual behavior (Sills, 1994, pp. 136-143). Those endorsing this view included police and correctional officers, insurance providers, physicians, corporate entities including the blood industry, and some segments of the public health community. This group came to the table with more institutional power and threatened to stop the adoption of any policy unless their concerns were met.

The police and correctional officers sought protection for workplace exposure including the ability to test without consent anyone whose blood they contacted. They also wanted criminal sanctions for the transmission of HIV and mandatory testing of all inmates coming into the state prison system. They urged the state to allow them to keep lists in their computer of suspected gay people within to ensure that they used appropriate precautions when responding to a scene. Insurance providers resisted any regulation or legislation that limited their ability to HIV test applicants for insurance (without their specific knowledge). They fought measures that would prohibit limitations on coverage for AIDS-related illnesses. The physicians wanted the ability to decline to treat anyone they should choose not to treat. They also wanted to limit their liability for failure to warn others of the HIV status of their patients.

Many large business entities wanted to ensure that the state did not enact regulations about employees with HIV. They urged more public sector care for people with HIV rather than relying on private insurance. Most of the large employers were self-insured and therefore were exempt from state regulation of insurance under ERISA.[11] ERISA provided little or no protection against discrimination in insurance coverage for people with HIV. The employers wanted the freedom to cap HIV coverage or choose not to provide coverage at all. At this time, the news media presented the President of Circle K, a convenience store corporation headquartered in Phoenix, sucking on his cigar and making a public announcement. He proudly stated that its self-insured health plan for Circle K employees would cover HIV-related infections as long as they were not caused by the acts of the individual. The plan did cover tobacco-related cancer. The national ACLU threatened a lawsuit. ERISA did not provide much of a legal ground to challenge this provision in the insurance plan. However, rather than defend such a suit, Circle K withdrew its restriction. The corporation's officers were present, however, when the Task Force began looking at how we could ensure that such provisions could be prevented in the future. They argued vehemently against any regulations that might affect them.

Large hospitals wanted complete discretion in their handling of infectious waste and treatment of HIV-infected employees and patients. They did not want the state regulating the ways that the hospital handled HIV-sensitive information in patient records. They resisted any efforts to enact laws that would create a cause of action for breach of confidentiality by a hospital employee. The blood services industry wanted to enhance blood shield laws to prevent liability for any transmission that occurred through the provision of blood. They urged anonymous testing because they believed that people were using the blood collection centers as a means to determine their HIV status to avoid by-name reporting. Finally, a small segment of the public health community wanted to put a quarantine procedure in place, require by-name reporting, and beef up contact tracing.

There were some issues that the entire Task Force embraced. These included the belief that education was one of the most effective tools in preventing the spread of HIV.[12] Many urged the State to adopt a policy of requiring education about HIV/AIDS of all nurses and physicians educated in the state as a condition of certification. The Task Force agreed that managed care was the most effective way to cope with the health needs of people with HIV. However, members disagreed about what "managed care" meant.

The members of the Task Force who saw their jobs as caring for people living with HIV had one advantage over the institutionally based faction. They had had more time during the planning process to devote to drafting recommendations.[13] Therefore, their language and perspectives colored the recommendations that were presented to the Task Force at the voting stage. We had expanded the membership of the Task Force to include two hundred additional (nonvoting) workers largely from community-based HIV support groups. They packed the public hearing room while the Task Force deliberated. This appeared to affect the formal membership. Nevertheless, those who perceived their job as "protecting the public" had more voting power on the Task Force. Consequently, the deliberations were long and difficult.

Many members of the Task Force argued that the recommendations that supported people with HIV "would not sell." They argued that innovative and costly ideas were good in theory but that we would be perceived as naive and "in the pocket" of people with HIV. This kind of argument makes it very easy not to grapple with the difficult policy choices that we had to make as a group. Many voting members objected to some language because they felt too identified with the document. No matter how little a role they had played in the drafting of the policy, they would be credited with authorship. Some policies would have extensive effect and significant financial consequences in the state. The simplest way of coping with their own accountability was to make decisions that were certain to be acceptable to others (Tetlock, 1985, p. 13). We could not afford to allow this concern to control our decision making since it would have required the Task Force to make no significant policy initiatives.

CONCLUSION: IMPLEMENTATION

The resulting policy initiatives reflect the tension between making hard policy choices and coping with public opinion. The Task Force Report recommended anonymous testing, civil rights protection for people with HIV, comprehensive education of children, education for health care providers and state employees, and other similar initiatives. It recommended funding more educational outreach programs for at-risk youth, women, and gay people. It urged the creation of an Office of Minority Health and Human Services to focus on minority health issues and increase minority participation in HIV/AIDS policy making.

The Task Force recommended that the State look into forming a risk pool insurance plan to cover its uninsurables. To increase the number of trained physicians, it recommended that the state establish a medical network of physicians and training program. The Task Force did not criticize the Public Health Department's failure to provide effective and culturally sensitive educational materials and resources to minority communities or gay men.[14] We retreated from a stand recommending regulations that would ensure insurance coverage for people with HIV as long as the insurance plan covered similar illnesses. We also withdrew from the recommendation that Arizona prisons provide condoms to incarcerated persons.

This consensus was the result of four grueling public meetings, each lasting approximately four hours and resulting in final votes. We published the result of our work in a 175-page book. Each recommendation clearly stated our position, the reason for that position, and the way to implement that recommendation. The Task Force closed, exhausted. We acted as if our work were done. In fact, it had just begun. Implementation was the key. The window of opportunity to see policy changes would remain open only a short while. Our work had generated a great deal of attention on the HIV issue. We needed to make those changes while that window was open.[15]

Governor Mofford extended the Task Force's life another year to monitor compliance with its recommendations. The public hearings throughout the state and the publication of the comprehensive report had made the chance for significant change more likely. Unfortunately, Task Force members had lost momentum. Most members, not personally affected by HIV, were tired of the issue. After over a year of consistent work on the Task Force Report, most of the members were content to go back to their full-time jobs. They trusted that the Governor's office would put the recommended executive acts in place. If an enterprising legislator wanted to initiate any legislation crafted as we suggested, then so be it. Fortunately, because we had been so inclusive of others in the community, there were people willing to follow through. They had not had the privilege nor the ordeal of working out agreement to the recommendations. The voting members of the Task Force delivered the document. Most of the HIV-activist community still had the energy to see the portions they favored enacted. Grass-roots organizations, fearing the discretionary nature of executive acts, moved forward to enact comprehensive legislation to ensure that many policies recommended by the Task Force had the force of law.

There were many aspects of the law that needed amending or whole sections that needed creating. This suggested a multitude of bills. Our Task Force experience taught us that people were reluctant to be connected to measures identified with people with HIV. We therefore chose an omnibus bill. The omnibus bill was over 20 pages long with amendments to many sections of the code and several new laws. Nearly all of the bill was written from the point of view of people with HIV. It included civil rights protection in employment and insurance and criminal penalties for breach of confidentiality. It protected workers from being precluded from claims for a workplace exposure. The bill prevented HIV testing without prior written consent in any circumstance. It required the state to offer anonymous testing. It required strict due process protection in the event the Department of Health exercised its quarantine powers.

Offering an omnibus bill rather than a plethora of separate bills was a "shoot the moon" kind of maneuver. We believed that the Legislature would vote it either up or down. No opponent to the bill would attempt to modify it for fear that they would become associated with the issue. Our guess was largely correct. The bill passed with very few modifications. This was due to three factors that I have identified: First, our guess that none would touch it because they might "get" AIDS was a very good call. Second, the lobbying opponents, like the medical association, corporate community, and the insurance industry, never believed the bill would pass. Therefore, they did not spend much energy on resisting it. Finally, our efforts as a Task Force to reach out to the community paid off. We mobilized a substantial number of citizens from all over the state to write and call their legislators and urge them to support the bill. We were also able to pack all hearing rooms on the bill with people who supported it.[16]

It has been several years since the bill passed, and since then, the institutional parties have had to take it seriously. It is the law. The result has been a systematic dismantling of each piece of the omnibus law.[17] Their task, however, has been much more difficult than ours. It is always harder to undo something that is done. Once the policy had been set in motion, it was difficult to stop. We had achieved much of what we wanted by the time opponents could mobilize their forces. We have also grown in our understanding of HIV and learned that it may be much better to mainstream HIV rather than create special rules for this disability.[18] State civil rights protection for people with HIV went a long way toward educating people that discrimination against people with HIV was illegal. The passage of the Americans with Disabilities Act did much to provide protection against discrimination. We have also become much more knowledgeable about the disease. That knowledge offsets the fear that prompted much of the discriminatory treatment in the past.

We had enormous obstacles and we were able to overcome some of them. This experience taught me that highly organized communities can affect policy making such that it offsets more institutionalized power. The only prerequisite is that the institutionalized power must either perceive no threat from the policy or be looking the other way. We were fortunate in Arizona to have dedicated people concerned about their community and willing to work very hard to be heard.

NOTES

1. This is not the person's real name. He has since died of HIV/AIDS, but despite the major violations of his privacy that occurred toward the end of his life, he remained a very private person.

2. In the last twenty years, anticipatory processes have become common and the simplest technique in a political environment is the "Futures Commission"–a process through which citizens analyze trends, develop alternative scenarios of the future, and establish recommendations and goals for the community (Osborne & Gaebler, 1993, p. 230).

3. According to the Centers for Disease Control, from June 1981 to September 1990, 152,126 cases of AIDS were reported to the U.S. Centers for Disease Control and although blacks constitute 12% of the population, they accounted for 28% of AIDS cases and the rate is increasing. Blacks also account for 73% of the total AIDS cases in heterosexual men, 52% in women, and 55% in children (Duh, 1991). Among Hispanics the rate of AIDS is almost three times that of the non-

Hispanic population. Hispanics accounted for 12.9% of the total number of cases nationally in 1981, and as of 1990 they constituted 15% of reported cases (Singer, Gonzalez, Vega, Centeno, & Davison, 1994, p. 59).

4. For more on Community-Based Organizations (CBOS) see Singer et al. (1994) and Altman (1994).

5. It was in a small working group of the Task Force that we first heard from Dana Mims, the produce worker mentioned at the beginning of the essay.

6. Again, I am using a fictitious name to protect the privacy of the individual.

7. Ultimately we achieved anonymous testing at the county test sites but not through private physicians.

8. For a discussion of the media and AIDS, see Lupton (1994).

9. This format was designed to create workable solutions that could be tested to determine if the goal was met. Osborne and Gaebler describe this process as strategic planning and have identified an eight-phase process. Their description is helpful in understanding the process that we went through as a Task Force and reduced to this recommendation format. The steps are as follows:
   1. analysis of the situation, both internal and external;
   2. diagnosis, or identification of the key issues;
   3. definition of mission;
   4. articulation of goals;
   5. creation of vision;
   6. development of strategy to realize the goals;
   7. development of a timetable;
   8. measurement of the results. (Osborne & Gaebler, 1993, p. 233)
Bryson (1988) provides a thorough introduction to the phases of strategic planning.

10. See Aiken (1987) and Freudenberg (1994, pp. 61-72) who discuss the impact of AIDS education and point out six obstacles to progress. The article by Freudenberg also discusses what future programs should comprise.

11. ERISA is a federal law that allows employers to provide their own benefit plans, including health insurance, subject to federal but not state regulation.

12. See Perrow and Guillen (1990, p. 25).

13. March and Olsen (1986, p. 21) suggest that people in a policy process do not have enough time to focus attention on particular things, nor can they spend too much time on one thing. Each person is faced with a personal decision on how much time to spend on a particular issue. As a result of the individual variations in the amount of time a person can allocate to an issue, some people have considerably more time to devote to decisions that are important to them. This affects the outcome of the policy or decision created.

14. Indeed, the problem of producing appropriate HIV educational materials plagues us today. Pedro Zamora, the young Cuban who played on MTV's *The Real World* and died November 11, 1994, was an advocate for educating people about AIDS. On July 12, 1994, he testified before the U.S. Congress asking for more explicit AIDS education programs. He said, "If you want to reach a young gay man, especially a young, gay man of color, then you need to give me information in the language and vocabulary I can understand and relate to" (*Boston*

Globe, November 12, 1994, Obituary, p. 25). Michal-Johnson and Bowen offer a chapter on HIV education that takes into account cultural experiences of those who are affected by HIV disproportionately. They argue that HIV education should focus on a cultural communication process as a means to prevent further spread of the disease (1992, pp. 147-192).

15. Kingdon (1984) describes the generation of alternatives and proposals in the community as the policy "primeval soup." In order to get those initiatives enacted, the policy community must be "softened up." As Kingdon puts it:

> To some degree ideas float freely through the policy primeval soup. But their advocates do not allow the process to be completely free-floating. In addition to starting discussions of their own proposals, they push their ideas in many different forums. They attempt to soften up both policy communities, which tend to be inertia-bound and resistant to major changes, and larger publics, getting them used to new ideas and building acceptance for their proposals. Then when a short-run opportunity to push the proposal comes, the way has been paved, the important people softened up. (p. 134)

16. For an in-depth analysis of different tactics of interest groups see Wilson (1981).

17. Since the passage of the law, a republican Governor has assumed power in Arizona and changed all of the heads of the relevant departments. This prevented many of the suggested changes in administrative policy from coming into effect. The insurance and medical associations have also successfully lobbied the legislature to delete sections of the AIDS Omnibus law that ensured many of the civil rights protection needs in the area of HIV.

18. See generally, Aiken and Musheno (1994).

REFERENCES

Aiken, J. H., & Musheno, M. (1994). Why Have-Nots Win in the HIV Litigation Arena: Socio-legal Dynamics of Extreme Cases. In M. Musheno (Ed.), "Special Issue on the Socio-legal Dynamics of AIDS" *Law and Policy, 16*(3).

Aiken, J. H. (1987). Education as Prevention. In H. L. Dalton & S. Burris (Eds.), *AIDS and the Law: A Guide for the Public* (pp. 90-105). New Haven, CT: Yale University Press.

Alford, R. (1975). *Health Care Politics.* Chicago: University of Chicago Press.

Altman, D. (1994). *Power and Community: Organizational and Cultural Response to AIDS.* Bristol, PA: Taylor & Francis.

Bayer, R., Levine, C., & Wolf, S. (1991). HIV Antibody Screening: An Ethical Framework for Evaluating Proposed Programs. In N. McKenzie (Ed.), *The AIDS Reader* (pp. 327-346). New York: Penguin Books.

Briathwaite, R., & Lythcott, N. (1991). Community Empowerment as a Strategy for Health Promotion for Black and Other Minority Populations. In N. McKenzie (Ed.), *The AIDS Reader* (pp. 522-533). New York: Penguin Books.

Bryson, J. M. (1988). *Strategic Planning for Public and Non Profit Organizations: A Guide to Strengthening and Sustaining Organizational Achievement*. San Francisco, CA: Jossey Bass, Inc., Publishers.

Duh, S. (1991). *Blacks and AIDS*. Newbury Park, CA: Sage.

Fox, D. M. (1988). AIDS and the American Health Polity: The History and Prospects of a Crisis of Authority. In E. Fee & D. Fox (Eds.), *AIDS: The Burdens of History* (pp. 316-343). Berkeley, CA: University of California Press.

Freudenberg, N. (1994). AIDS Prevention in the United States: Lessons from the First Decade. In N. Krieger & G. Margo (Eds.), *AIDS: The Politics of Survival*. Amityville, NY: Baywood Publishing.

Osborne, D., & Gaebler, T. (1993). *Reinventing Government: How the Entrepreneurial Spirit Is Transforming the Public Sector*. New York: Penguin Books.

Kingdon, J. W. (1984). *Agendas, Alternatives, and Public Policies*. Michigan: Harper Collins.

Lupton, D. (1994). *Moral Threats and Dangerous Desires: AIDs in the News Media*. Bristol, PA: Taylor & Francis.

March, J. G., & Olsen, J. P. (1986). Garbage Can Models of Decision Making in Organizations. In J. G. March & R. Wissinger-Baylor (Eds.), *Ambiguity and Command: Organizational Perspectives on Military Decision Making* (p. 21).

Michal-Johnson, P., & Bowen, S. (1992). The Place of Culture in HIV Education. T. Edgar, M. Fitzpatrick, & V. Freimuth (Eds.), In *AIDS: A Communication Perspective*. Hillsdale, NJ: Lawrence Erlbaum Associates, Inc.

Perrow, C., & Guillen, M. (1990). *The AIDS Disaster*. New Haven, CT: Yale University Press.

Shilts, R. (1987). *And the Band Played On*. New York: St. Martin's Press.

Sills, Y. G. (1994). *The AIDS Pandemic*. Westport, CT: Greenwood Press.

Singer, M., Gonzalez, W., Vega, E., Centeno, I., & Davison, L. (1994). Implementing a Community Based AIDS Prevention Program for Ethnic Minorities: The Comunidad y Responsibilidad Project. In J. Van Vugt (Ed.), *AIDS Prevention and Services: Community Based Research*. Westport, CT: Bergin & Garvey.

Tetlock, P. E. (1985). Accountability: The Neglected Social Context of Judgment and Choice. In *Research in Organizational Behavior*. New York: JAI Press. Vol 7.

Wilson, G. (1981). *Interest Groups in the United States*. Oxford: Clarendon.

AIDS and the New Medical Gaze: Bio-Politics, AIDS, and Homosexuality

Dion Dennis, PhD

Texas A & M International University

SUMMARY. The essay argues that the contemporary resurgence of homophobia and the remedicalization of homosexuals in the wake of AIDS is, in part, an unintended but predictable effect of a quarter century of fractious identity-politics. Prominent gay and lesbian political strategies of the 1970s and 1980s borrowed heavily from increasingly discredited, if once politically correct, discourses that valorized individuals on the basis of membership in governmentally constructed bio-bureaucratic categories. Drawing on the work of prominent gay intellectuals, such as Foucault, Watney, and Richard Rodriguez, and locating their insights within the context of contemporary cultural and political conflicts, the essay argues that gay advocates who essentialize homosexual identity, however benignly, unwittingly participate in constituting the ground for an emergence of a neoeugenic movement at millennium's end. The essay concludes with the observation that escaping the conceptual prison of bio-bureaucratic categories is not a uniquely gay or lesbian task. It is a human task. *[Article copies available for a fee from The Haworth Document Delivery Service: 1-800-342-9678. E-mail address: getinfo@haworth. com]*

Dion Dennis is Assistant Professor at Texas A & M International University. Correspondence may be addressed: Department of Criminal Justice, History, Political Science and Geography, Texas A & M International University, 5201 University Blvd., Laredo, TX 78041-1499 [E-mail address: ddennis@icsi.net.].

[Haworth co-indexing entry note]: "AIDS and the New Medical Gaze: Bio-Politics, AIDS, and Homosexuality." Dennis, Dion. Co-published simultaneously in *Journal of Homosexuality* (The Haworth Press, Inc.) Vol. 32, No. 3/4, 1997, pp. 169-184; and: *Activism and Marginalization in the AIDS Crisis* (ed: Michael A. Hallett) The Haworth Press, Inc., 1997, pp. 169-184; and: *Activism and Marginalization in the AIDS Crisis* (ed: Michael A. Hallett) Harrington Park Press, an imprint of The Haworth Press, Inc., 1997, pp. 169-184. Single or multiple copies of this article are available for a fee from The Haworth Document Delivery Service [1-800-342-9678, 9:00 a.m. - 5:00 p.m. (EST). E-mail address: getinfo@haworth.com].

> My subject is not the truth of being but the social being of truth, not whether facts are real but what the politics of their representation are. My aim is to release what he noted as the enormous energy of history that lies bonded [in popular taken-for-granted narratives]. The history that showed things "as they really were," [Walter Benjamin] pointed out, was the strongest narcotic of our century. And of course, it still is. (Taussig, 1987)

One can understand the hankering, common among some gay activists and their allies, for a respite from the ceaseless and peripatetic local, national, and global wars of identity-politics that have been fought over the last quarter-century. Some battles have been won. Others have been lost. Some, like the status of gays in the military, remain as active sites of ongoing legal and cultural confrontation. And in highly complex venues, like the tragic and paradoxical effects of the AIDS epidemic, definitions of gain and loss have become distressingly muddy, polyvalent, and contingent. And, after the political and cultural struggles of a quarter-century, feelings of vulnerability and potential disenfranchisement remain as intense and as valid as ever. For that which has been undeniably gained seems forever consigned to the zone of the contested and contestable. But in all the flux of shifting bodies, rhetoric, and politics, another constant remains. That is, the ambiguities, multiplicities, and sheer rhizomic diversity of gay and lesbian identities exceed any attempt to define and domesticate the expressive range of what it means to be gay or lesbian (or human, put in the broadest possible context). But in bureaucratic social and political fields where the effective exercise of power compels the prefabrication of self-identical and demonstrably well organized representations of constituencies with clout, a classic conundrum emerges. Arlene Stein puts it this way:

> The paradox is that if we don't name our difference in explicitly sexual terms, we remain invisible as lesbians–but if we do name it we're typecast as little more than sexual beings, and the vast complexity of our lives disappears. (Berman, citing Stein, 1993)

This is an unpleasant Catch-22 that spurs acts of symbolic guerilla politics from gay groups that are designed to destabilize such binarisms. For example, Rosemary Coombe recounts that

> In Toronto one day, pedestrians were surprised to see the following message flashing on an electronic billboard: "Lesbians Fly Air Canada," it repeatedly flashed. The next day the message was gone. A gay rights group had broadcast the statement to remind people of the similarities between lesbians and all other Canadians by evoking the archetypal "normal" Canadian experience. [This] stopped when Air Canada threatened to apply for an injunction to stop the group from using its name. (Coombe, 1991)

The late Randy Shilts's oft-repeated comment that a biological explanation for homosexuality "would reduce being gay to something like being left-handed" reflects a similar integrationist desire to be regarded as "normal." It is a bid to defuse the symbolic politics of identity and difference around "sexual orientation" to a stylistic margin. Such a benign margin would presumably be mutually and pleasantly inhabited by the designers of left-handed doorknobs and consumer products for gays and lesbians. Missing from Shilts's wistful comment is the Foucauldian insight that *all* bodies have become busy matrices invested with power and knowledge relations in Euro-Western societies.

Joe Sartelle, in a recent article examining several strands of popular gay essentialism, describes how Texas journalist Molly Ivins, in a December 1993 column, constructs her gay essentialism. Ivins's narrative starts with a series of Shilts-like assertions:

> Homosexuality is not a choice. It is a human condition, fixed before one becomes sexually active. It cannot be changed by will. No one chooses to be homosexual any more than people choose to be heterosexual or brown-eyed or left-handed. (Sartelle, citing Ivins, 1994)

From this dictum, Ivins then collapses the diversity of gay identity by subsequently prattling on about the famous drag queens of Richardson County, Texas. By doing so, Ivins reinforces the deplorably over-determined image of gays and lesbians as gender inverts. That is, "they" are all effeminate men and butch women. By doing so, Ivins is witlessly participating and reinforcing the very poverty-struck representations of "normal" and "abnormal" sexuality that police desire, expression, and the imaginative limits of possible heterosexual, bisexual, and homosexual identities. That is, both Shilts and Ivins are naive. And their sloppy, unreflective biologically flavored thinking on sexual desire, behavior, and identity is potentially dangerous. As writers on eugenics (Kelves, 1985), anthropology (Gould, 1981), and current designer genetics (Lewontin, 1992) show over and over again, all biological paradigms, eminent and infamous, are inherently ideological products. They are, in significant part, the complex effects of the social, cultural, and political orders from which they emerge. That is, biology as social ideology in practice is enmeshed in everyday discourse and the circulating regimes of commercial and noncommercial signs. Bio-ideology is coded into the nondiscursive operation of machines and the functions of architecture. It shapes the protocols and rules that fund research and public service. In all these cases and more, we would do well to recall Simon Watney's words on the relation between biological activities and the symbolic construction of communities.

> It is up to us to define the terms in which [the scandal of AIDS treatment] will be eventually understood. This involves a commitment to the fullest possible understanding of the ways in which the psychic reality of all aspects of human sexuality are always organized symbolically in excess of both biological needs and the demands of many cultural and political roles that sexuality is currently used to naturalize and legitimate. AIDS demonstrates the *practical* need to insist upon a non-naturalistic explanation of *all* adult sexuality. (Watney, 1989)

HOMOSEXUALS AS DANGEROUS, HOMOSEXUALS IN DANGER: DANGER AND THE BIRTH OF THE HOMOSEXUAL

We're going to have a society of dangers, with, on the one side, those who are in danger and, on the other, those who are dangerous. And sexuality will be a kind of roaming danger, a sort of omnipresent phantom. Sexuality will become a threat in all social relations. And what we will have is a new regime for the supervision of sexuality; in the second half of the 20th Century it may be decriminalized, but only to [re]appear in the form of a universal danger. I'd say that [that is the danger]. (Foucault, 1988)

Throughout much of his work, the late Michel Foucault focused on the emergence of key "dividing practices" by which human subjectivities were interdependently constituted as objects of knowledge and subjects of power. In detail, Foucault has shown how the emerging choreography of institutional procedures and forms (the prison, school, hospital, army, asylum) are linked, directly and indirectly, with the deployment and expansion of specific types of knowledges. A basic feature of the human sciences (which Foucault once termed "the political anatomy of detail") from the eighteenth century to the present, are objectivizing practices that constitute many of the taken-for-granted categories (and boundaries) between "the mad and the sane, the sick and the healthy, the criminal and the good." These categories (and the development of statistical methods that engendered vast administrative bureaucracies) emerged as the industrial revolution spurred an exponential growth in poor, destitute, and mobile urban populations. These categories and statistical methodologies gave birth to techniques of specific and general prevention. That is, this was also the advent of statistical regimes of risk-management (such as insurance technology and epidemiology).

Foucault termed this phenomenon, this organization of human life as the prime object of knowledge for the emerging disciplines, *bio-power* (Foucault, 1990). Bio-power consists of detailed and rationalized administrative procedures designed to optimize and control human "life" along the twin goals of maximal economic productivity and political docility. The dual poles of bio-power that take life as an object of knowledge are an "anatomo-politics of the human body" and "a bio-politics of a population." The former deals with the breakdown and detailed retraining of a given body to achieve an identity/skill nexus. (The "basic training" used to turn a homeboy into a soldier in "boot camp" is a good example of "anatomo-politics.") The latter, the "bio-politics of the population," refers to the regulation and administration of populations along general and specific demographic axes. (These include birth and mortality rates, public health, migratory patterns, and ethnic composition. These now include such things as marketing data in the form of consumption patterns, attitudes, and behaviors.) Caught in the cross hairs between the disciplines of the body and the management of populations is the political question of sexuality. As a "case" in a population, it is situated at the intersection of the two poles of bio-power. For Foucault, notions of sex and sexuality, as repression and liberation, are the historical products of nineteenth century "dividing practices" (of the normative and the pathological) and do not represent "the truth of being." They are part of the social being of truth, part of the politics of representation to be found in current regimes of bio-power.

During the last quarter of the nineteenth century, criminological anthropologists and psychiatrists (often one and the same) promulgated psycho-medical analyses of criminality and homosexuality. Subjects that committed these acts were often characterized as "abnormal" human types, the bearers of pathologies shaped by genetic (eugenic), psychological, and social forces. Generally, these bio-typologies depicted "criminals" and "homosexuals" as weak and unable to inhibit acting on their inherently "degenerate" impulses. That is, because of how their identities were constituted within these frameworks, as pathological genetic specimens, they were described as having "little or no choice." These bio-analyses became a point of departure, in penal and psychological practice, for a class of professionals, trained in the medical gaze, to invent the procedures and detailed classification schemata that became the backbone of psychiatric evaluation. These crypto-analyses are the origins of the classification of "the homosexual" as a pathology in the *Diagnostic and Statistical Manual,* Versions 1 & 2 (DSM I, DSM II) of the American Psychological Association (APA). In short, both criminality and homosexuality ceased being primarily defined by specific acts of behavior. Criminality and homosexuality became the decipherable signs of innate bio-attributes of identity.

Homo criminalis and *homo sexualis* were species that could be found under the overarching genus of "The Dangerous Individual."

As Watney notes, gay culture in the 1970s took major steps in forging non-essentialist social identities sturdy and secure enough to successfully contest restrictive and stigmatizing forms of institutional practice in medical, social, and legal venues. In 1980, at the onset of the AIDS epidemic, the APA, in its (then) new DSM-III, removed homosexuality from its definitive laundry list of reimbursable pathologies. It has since become a painful and bitter irony, therefore, that at the moment that gay identity was medically depathologized (dehomosexualized) that the AIDS epidemic would provide a vehicle for sustained cultural and political attempts to secure a repathologization, a rehomosexualization of gay identity under the gaze of medical, moral, and theological institutions, texts, and "authorities." For like *scientia sexualis* itself, the representation-effects of the AIDS epidemic lie squarely at the intersection of "the life of the [individual] body and the life of the species." And though "danger" has never been a medico-psychiatric category, it is a flexible political signifier *par excellence*. Representations of "danger" have become prolific at the twilight of progressive capitalism. In a time of economic decline and eroding political sovereignty that is characterized by escalating regimes of privatized security and harsh class polarization, evocations of the dangerous are extremely potent. Deprived of the bipolarity of the Cold War,

> The war machine finds its new object as a function of the real, very special kind of peace it promotes and has already installed. It no longer needs a qualified enemy but operates against the "unspecified enemy," domestic or foreign (an individual, group, class, people, event, world). There arises from this new conception of security as materialized war, as organized insecurity or molecularized, distributed, programmed catastrophe. (Deleuze & Guattari, 1987)

That is, the "enemy" must be invented, vanquished, and then reincarnated. For "the enemy" is a projected space of untameable darkness, murky chaos, and unspeakable excess of unfathomable "Otherness." This production of "Otherness" is how societies constitute themselves as domesticated, self-identical, and knowable sites. In a paradoxical time where economic and informational globalization is paired with heightened expressions and acts of ethnic or site-based territoriality, much of U.S. political life has been marked by a shifting allocation of attention to "unspecified enemies." In the last few years, "we" (which is itself an "unspecified homogeneity") have constituted a plethora of "enemies." A few, among others, are Noriega, Saddam Hussein, the Japanese economic-will-to-power, Haitian refugees, Mexican economic migrants, North Korea, "crime" (which itself is a key signifier of known but unspecified enemies), governmental spending, bureaucratic regulation, welfare recipients, and inner-city gangs. According to Sidney Blumenthal,

> In America, as in Europe, the [dissolution of the Evil Empire, the Soviet Union] unleashed ethnic and religious tensions that had been mostly submerged for nearly half a century. Pat Buchanan's call at the [1992 Republican Convention] for "cultural warfare" was an instance of such post-Cold War atavism. The old dichotomies are breaking down. There are some ideological categories that have no history in the politics of the Cold War. The ends of wars bring chaos and recriminations [and] are periods of enormous [political] realignment. (Blumenthal, 1994)

But while signifiers of dangerousness seem fluid and recodable (hence "unspecified"), there are evocative problematics that serve as recurrent "strange attractors" for social movements. Some of the fiercest contestations revolve around the specific formulation and subsequent policing of "dividing practices"–legal/criminal, moral/immoral and normal/pathological–along reproductive and sexual axes. As noted earlier, these disputed practices (such as abortion, needle distribution to IV drug users, sex and AIDS education, euthanasia, genetic screenings and therapies, the dispensing of condoms to teenagers, and homosexuality) meet at the nexus of practices of self-care with the administration of the populace. And the once simplistic racial and ethnic formulas for the administration of the populace has itself been complicated, in a time of rapid demographic transformations, by a prolific expansion of separatist claims to a privileged minority status. And, in some sense, Evangelical nativist discourse, expressed by the Reverend Lou Sheldon, Chairman of the Traditional Values Coalition (TVC), that states

> We were here first. You don't take our shared common values and say they are biased and bigoted . . . We are the keepers of what is right and wrong. (Blumenthal, 1994)

is itself a response to marginalization, by poor or downwardly mobile whites. According to Richard Rodriguez,

> Here in California we are headed for trouble. The state is filled with minorities–Guatemalans, West Hollywood gays, Chinese immigrants, senior citizens, religious fundamentalists. We are an Alice in Wonderland state where the majority of us claim to be minorities.
>
> I think about skinheads. Hateful, angry, mean as snakes. They know they do not count in America. Literally do not count. They have been written out of the civil rights agenda for the last 30 years because they are white. (Rodriguez, 1994)

If I understand Rodriguez (a classically educated, middle-aged, bronze-skinned gay man brought up by Irish Catholic nuns) aright, *then the resurgence of homophobic and racist groups such as skinheads is, in part, an unintended but predictable effect of a quarter-century of identity-politics that valorizes **who people are** in terms of the artifices of bio-bureaucratic categories,* rather than attending to more salient, less racially tinged features such as social class, education, or degrees of poverty and marginalization. According to Lawrence Wright,

> Washington [D.C.] in the millennial years is a city of warring racial and ethnic groups fighting for recognition, protection and entitlements. How much this contest has widened, how bitter it has turned, how complex and baffling it is, and how far-reaching its consequences are became evident in a series of congressional hearings that concluded in November, 1993. (Wright, 1994)

Insofar as *some* organized gay and lesbian groups unreflexively deploy the rhetoric and bureaucratic tactics of a so-called "progressive" racial politics, a corruptible politics that is increasingly in ruins as a just or workable model for entitlements, *a gay politics of freedom may be swept up by an impending turn-of-the-century political repudiation of ersatz bio-essentialist constructions of race, ethnicity, and gender.* As Kelves (1985), Hacking (1991), Foucault (1978, 1990), Said (1978), and others have pointedly shown, the construction and subsequent identification of the Self with a rigid field of predetermined categories emerged from nineteenth century projects of imperial and industrial administration (domestic and colonial). But in the rapidly accelerating disjunctures of race, place, class, and ethnicity in the New World (Dis)Order, the initial rudimentary binary divisions (of race, class, gender, and sexual orientation) have become destabilized along dual poles. First, the polarities have been reversed. Since the 1960s, a set of attributes that were valorized now stand as stereotypical objects of derision. For example: To assert, in the political climate of the U.S. universities, that someone is "a white, middle-aged, heterosexual, Euro-centric male" is a de facto politically correct form of bigotry (after Rodriguez, 1994). That is, the structural dynamics of valorization and marginalization continue. But those that are ostracized inherit mechanisms that sustain and promote powerful economies of grievance. And these are the structural positions now held by (among others) the increasingly well organized Christian right, anti-abortion groups, and skinheads.

Secondly, the invention and aggressive advancement of bio-political categories has been rhizomic. That is, as Rodriguez says, California is "where the majority claims to be minority" (Rodriguez, 1994). According to Wright, because increasingly capricious differences of pigmentation and lineage determine the dispersion of a lucrative array of entitlements, a harsh zero-sum identity-game now dominates ethnic politics. And these deadly contests are simultaneously enacted in the halls of government and on the streets of urban barrios and ghettos that serve as de facto war zones (Martinez, 1994).

As a form of a bio-politics of the body, as a bio-politics of representation, gay politics is deeply enmeshed in these other forms of bodies and their representation. In my estimation, the danger for gay politics is in the potential failure to recognize and avoid such bio-political snares. In bad scenes, like the one below, polarities may be reversed but key dichotomies endure undisturbed while hate and the will-to-dominate flourish.

In Kendall County, Texas (1994), a militant middle-aged white male, a member of Pat Robertson's Christian Coalition, runs for a position on the local school board in an affluent suburb of San Antonio, Texas. We see and hear him on KSAT News. Agitated, he pledges to tirelessly work to suppress homosexuality in the schools, conflating it with criminality and Satanism. Meanwhile, on another San Antonio station, his 25-year-old daughter, A., appears on *Geraldo*. She is a large leather lesbian who works as a heterosexual dominatrix in the Oak Lawn district of Dallas. In private conversations, she utters her unqualified loathing for all men. Mistress Marie, as she is known to her clientele of well-to-do slaves, regards "the male" as contemptible and as an inherently degenerative biological form (personal conversation, Roxana Zapata, 1994).

These dual subject-positions, father and daughter, inhabit the same essentialist structure of knowledge and identity. Together, they reproduce the standard discourse of valorization and marginalization. It is only the polarities that are reversed. Each needs the other to sustain an economic and bio-political identity. Together, the patriarch, zealous in his quest for a Christian Reich, and his daughter, eager to act out the dark underside of that vision upon the flesh of paying male slaves, are locked in a death dance. It is the hegemony of the technical practices of bio-power, attached to a certain quasi-morality, that produces such unhappy results. And it is to these that we now turn.

BIOCRACY AND THE BID FOR A CHRISTIAN REICH: POSSIBLE DIRECTIONS FOR GAY POLITICS AT MILLENNIUM'S END

In an earlier section, Foucault predicted that sexuality would be recoded "in the form of a universal danger." One vivid example is below. The following is an excerpt from Pat Robertson's *700 Club* (on CBN) for the week of March 1, 1993:

Pat: [School-based sex education] is a dangerous steam roller that's going to destroy families in America. It's going to destroy the lives of innocent little children, because they're not ready. I mean they ought to be allowed to play, and have dolls, or choo-choo trains. They should be ALLOWED TO DEVELOP without sexuality being forced upon them by these deviants.

A magazine called Sexology [is] behind this. They are anti-family, anti-God, anti-traditional values, and they want to open up our children to all kinds of bizarre sex, and it's WRONG. They say we can't have Bibles in the school, we can't let the kids pray, but we're training them how to be homosexuals. (Robertson, 1993)

In all its stages, the educational apparatus is a key site of bio-power. It works to create productive and docile subjects. But there are struggles over the type of desirable minds and bodies that the technology of the school should produce. And Robertson's commentary, which was folded into a CBN news report on the status of a sex education program in Georgia's schools, is but one site of struggle. For gay politics, the importance of Robertson's tirade unfolds along several tracks. First, Robertson conflates ALL school-based sex education as the dangerous work of generic "deviants," an ad hominem argument that is imbued with the rhetorical normative authority accorded to the medical gaze. Secondly, all sex education is constituted as inherently "anti-family, anti-God, anti-traditional values." With this move, Robertson fashions his claim as pro-family, pro-God, and pro-traditional values, nobly defending innocent children from perverted sexologists. Thirdly, if all non-Evangelically approved sex education is "bizarre" (that is, abnormal to the Biblically normative gazer), then all those who teach sex education must be "training them [children] how to be homosexuals." This series of rhetorical maneuvers climaxes with the figure of the "abnormal" homosexual as the penultimate "anti-Christ" and as a Satanic signifier. It is meant as the intolerable cap on a panoply of disgusting tactics perpetrated on children, families, and God. In the Robertsonian universe, this is the dreaded result to which all sex education programs are held equally culpable.

In notable ways, how Robertson and other Christian Fascists shape discourses and practices of homophobia parallels Edward Said's portrait of European cultural and academic forms of Orien-

Index

NOTES: Reference sources and author names are selectively indexed, primarily only when full titles and names are cited in text.

The *Foreword* is not indexed.

End-of-chapter Notes and text footnotes are selectively indexed, and indicated by "n" and "fn" respectively.

Page series preceded by *mentioned* indicates subject is intermittently discussed on all inclusive pages.

Page numbers in *italics* denote illustrations.

Square brackets [ ] denote information provided by indexer.

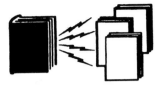

Haworth
DOCUMENT DELIVERY
SERVICE

This valuable service provides a single-article order form for any article from a Haworth journal.

- *Time Saving:* No running around from library to library to find a specific article.
- *Cost Effective:* All costs are kept down to a minimum.
- *Fast Delivery:* Choose from several options, including same-day FAX.
- *No Copyright Hassles:* You will be supplied by the original publisher.
- *Easy Payment:* Choose from several easy payment methods.

Open Accounts Welcome for . . .
- Library Interlibrary Loan Departments
- Library Network/Consortia Wishing to Provide Single-Article Services
- Indexing/Abstracting Services with Single Article Provision Services
- Document Provision Brokers and Freelance Information Service Providers

---

MAIL or *FAX* THIS ENTIRE ORDER FORM TO:

Haworth Document Delivery Service
The Haworth Press, Inc.
10 Alice Street
Binghamton, NY 13904-1580

or FAX: 1-800-895-0582
or CALL: 1-800-342-9678
9am-5pm EST

PLEASE SEND ME PHOTOCOPIES OF THE FOLLOWING SINGLE ARTICLES:

1) Journal Title: _____
   Vol/Issue/Year: _____ Starting & Ending Pages: _____
   Article Title: _____
   _____

2) Journal Title: _____
   Vol/Issue/Year: _____ Starting & Ending Pages: _____
   Article Title: _____
   _____

3) Journal Title: _____
   Vol/Issue/Year: _____ Starting & Ending Pages: _____
   Article Title: _____
   _____

4) Journal Title: _____
   Vol/Issue/Year: _____ Starting & Ending Pages: _____
   Article Title: _____
   _____

(See other side for Costs and Payment Information)

COSTS: Please figure your cost to order quality copies of an article.

1. Set-up charge per article: $8.00

               ($8.00 × number of separate articles)   _____

2. Photocopying charge for each article:

               1-10 pages: $1.00   _____

               11-19 pages: $3.00   _____

               20-29 pages: $5.00   _____

               30+ pages: $2.00/10 pages   _____

3. Flexicover (optional): $2.00/article   _____

4. Postage & Handling: US: $1.00 for the first article/

               $.50 each additional article   _____

               Federal Express: $25.00   _____

               Outside US: $2.00 for first article/

               $.50 each additional article _____

5. Same-day FAX service: $.35 per page   _____

                      GRAND TOTAL: _____

METHOD OF PAYMENT: (please check one)

❑ Check enclosed   ❑ Please ship and bill. PO # _____
                         (sorry we can ship and bill to bookstores only! All others must pre-pay)

❑ Charge to my credit card: ❑ Visa; ❑ MasterCard; ❑ Discover;
                          ❑ American Express;

Account Number: _____ Expiration date: _____

Signature: ✗ _____

Name: _____ Institution: _____

Address: _____

_____

City: _____ State: _____ Zip: _____

Phone Number: _____ FAX Number: _____

MAIL or *FAX* THIS ENTIRE ORDER FORM TO:

Haworth Document Delivery Service | **or FAX:** 1-800-895-0582
The Haworth Press, Inc. | **or CALL:** 1-800-342-9678
10 Alice Street | 9am-5pm EST)
Binghamton, NY 13904-1580

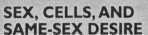

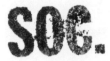